Dr T
....

Dr T

A Guide to Sexual Health and Pleasure

....

Dr Tlaleng Mofokeng (MBChB)

To Minda,

May this book bring
you joy.
To Big O's and
    Revolutionary Pleasure.

MACMILLAN

Dr T

Every effort has been made to ensure the accuracy of the medical
information and advice contained in this book, but the onus is on
the reader to consult with a medical professional to verify and clarify
anything that he or she is not sure of. Remember that Google is not
a doctor!

First published in 2019 by Pan Macmillan South Africa
Private Bag X19,
Northlands
Johannesburg
2116

www.panmacmillan.co.za

ISBN 978-1-77010-646-8
eISBN 978-1-77010-647-5

Editing by Jane Bowman
Proofreading by Claire Heckrath
Design and typesetting by Triple M Design
Illustrations sourced from iStock
Cover design by publicide
Author photographs by Zuzi Seoka
Make-up by Nikki Pitso
Hair by Unathi Ntakana

Me,

You,

Us.

Our lives

Our herstory

Our sexualities

Our experiences

You and I

Us.

We are!

The Indomitable.

Contents

Section 2: Sexual Pleasure

Section 3: Sexual Rights

Introduction

....

'Please be advised that the following feature is a PG16 due to the sexual content' is the introduction 'disclaimer' I now open with! At the start of almost all my radio sexual health segments I contribute to, this is the tagline I have become accustomed to but I definitely didn't ever think it would be.

In 2010, two years after graduating from medical school, I was working in the West Rand townships, on the outskirts of Johannesburg. As a response to the HIV epidemic, there was a public campaign across the country and the district I was working in was one of the hubs of activity to get more peer educators enrolled into a HIV prevention programme for the local community. This was at a time when our country, South Africa, was engaged in finding more creative ways of accessing the youth and getting them to sign up to do voluntary HIV testing. Much was being said about reducing risky behaviour and it was still very technical in its approach by ways of risk reduction in wider public health campaigns. Clinics were labelled 'youth-friendly' but there was not much focus on training a new crop of healthcare professionals who could incorporate sexuality, gender and sexual pleasure in the consultations with young people.

As a young 20-something-old, even I, with all the medical knowledge, felt that the approach that was being used, stigmatised young people having sex and sex became something looked at as inherently diseased. This feeling was not just a feeling. Once I started doing research I found that many healthcare providers do not talk with their adolescent patients about sexual health issues during primary care visits. When these conversations do occur, they are usually very brief; in one study conversations with patients aged 12 to 17 lasted an average of 36 seconds.

By the end of the first few months of working at the clinic as the resident medical officer, I noticed there were more young women and men waiting in the car park for me than there were in the clinic. The conversations we started having were casual. None of them were acutely ill so once the initial 'icebreaking' was done, we swiftly move on and chatted about girlfriends and boyfriends, how to break up with someone, how to say no to sex when you feel you are not ready, sexual pleasure, what the different parts of the vulva are and the list goes on! A young woman asked me if it was true that masturbation caused one to lose the ability to be sexual and to have pleasurable sex in the future. Another asked if it was normal to have vaginal dryness. Their preference for the car park consultations persisted for as long as I worked at the clinic and became something I looked forward to. I often joke and say I'm not sure when exactly I became the sex doctor but those young people had a big part to play in what has become my life's work.

I do not recall ever feeling awkward or shy to talk about sex or sexual health-related topics and for that I have my mother to credit. She was always open about sex and relationships and would often have 'sex talks' in a very nonchalant manner. She made me comfortable with my own sexuality and thus the ability to share knowledge in a non-judgemental manner. Those young people felt comfortable talking to me about their sexual health and because I looked like them, I spoke like them and I used the same slang as they did, it was easy for them to connect with me.

I found myself at the end of my contract with the clinic and realised I had to find a way to reach as many young people as I could. I needed to be able to reach them where they were at any given time and research has shown that digital media, including social networking sites, apps and text messaging services are increasingly being used to reach adolescents with sexual health interventions, and studies have demonstrated efficacy in improving knowledge and behaviour across a range of sexual health outcomes. In South Africa, recent data shows that digital media and access to mobile phones is growing exponentially, with an expected mobile internet penetration of 52.3% in 2016 with figures set to increase to 77.8% in 2021.

So this is how my journey started; with a cellphone and mobile data. I was soon contributing as a sexual health expert across multiple platforms such as radio, television, print and social media, on both a local and global scale. My Twitter account today is constantly buzzing with requests for information and referrals for sexual and reproductive care services. And I also contribute to *The Sunday Times* and have been published in a range of media houses including *The Guardian*, *Cosmopolitan* SA, *Teen Vogue*, Women24 and am the resident sexual health expert on one of the top three biggest national radio stations, Metro FM, with a previous weekly slot at the regional station, KayaFM, for three years.

It is not always easy knowing how to measure the impact of an initiative, working alone, mostly on digital platforms, but what started off as an extramural activity quickly became a recognisable brand of health communication. In 2016, I was given an award by the Bill and Melinda Gates Foundation, the 120 Under 40: The New Generation of Family Planning Leaders, for my work as a health communicator. And in 2017 I was invited to partake in a webinar hosted by the Johns Hopkins Bloomberg School of Public Health, where I shared my experiences and the ways I use digital media to build a strong brand in the public health field. It meant so much being recognised by my peers for the value of my work.

In 2018, I expanded to becoming host and associate producer of a television show 'Sex Talk with Dr T' on the Moja Love channel on DSTV. I embarked on the project to showcase what sex positivity looks like as well as to bring evidence-based and inclusive programming, while being deliberate in ensuring inclusion of gender and sexualities beyond the heteronormative. The educational aspect of the edutainment covered topics such as sex work decriminalisation and interviewing sex worker advocacy groups on human rights law, health and law reform.

My approach and goal is to elevate sexual pleasure to its rightful place alongside sexual health and sexual rights. Another platform that I use is on a podcast entitled 'PodSexEd' which is a series of conversations between myself and a friend where we discuss issues such as menstrual hygiene, sex toys, our experiences within the feminist/advocacy spaces and dedicate entire episodes to the clitoris and discussions around pleasure and masturbation. My weekly Q and A column in *The Sunday Times* also reaches thousands of people, via a more 'traditional' platform.

One of the most common negative comments I receive in terms of my work is whether we are making it easy for young people to have sex. A large body of research has found no evidence that providing young people with sexual and reproductive health information and education results in increased sexual risk-taking. In fact, comprehensive life skills-based sexuality education helps young people gain the knowledge and skills to make conscious, healthy and respectful choices about relationships and sexuality.

And as such, recommended by the American College of Obstetricians and Gynecologists' Committee on Adolescent Health Care, advocacy programmes should not only focus on reproductive development, the prevention of STIs, and unintended pregnancy, but they also should teach about forms of sexual expression, healthy sexual and nonsexual relationships, gender identity and sexual orientation and questioning, communication, recognising and preventing sexual violence, consent, and decision making.

It is with this in mind that my work is dedicated to ensuring that programmes and health systems link sexual health, sexual rights and sexual pleasure and to translate this into sex positive communication and access to inclusive sexual healthcare in order to support young people make healthy transitions into adulthood.

Dr T
Johannesburg
June 2019

About this book

∙∙∙

I wrote this book, A *Guide to Sexual Health and Pleasure*, with the inten-tion of helping you, the reader, navigate different aspects of sexual and reproductive health, pleasure and rights. The experiences I have had as a young woman, the many conversations I've had with women, specifi-cally my mother, Ausi Aggie, my medical training, as well the 12 years of practice, have all prepared me for this moment.

I draw on and find the courage to be myself from my experiences with my mother. I am truly only able to do this work, confidently and boldly, because of the way my mother affirmed my inquisitiveness as a child. She taught me vital life lessons and gave me information about sex, relationships and my body, in a way that made me trust her as a resource. But I realised growing up that not all young people had a care-giver or parent who was as affirming, delicate and informative as my mother was to me and so I hope this book is a resource for many young people, caregivers, parents and anyone working with young people. My aim is to promote wellness in order to achieve the maximal point pos-sible for pleasure.

The first section of the book, Sexual Health, deals with health and wellness and covers common medical conditions and provides infor-mation to assist you in understanding your own anatomy and bodily functions. You may be interested in a certain aspect because of a per-sonal connection or because you have always wondered about certain anatomy or a specific illness. Whatever your reason or interest, the section provides all the details which, once understood, will alleviate anxiety caused by simply not knowing. It busts some common myths by providing accurate information to assist in making informed decisions about your health and pleasure.

The second section, Sexual Pleasure, is a dedication to the Pleasure Revolution. Sexual pleasure is the missing link in many sexual health discussions and even in the medical field, women's pleasure is under-researched, with the development for safe and effective pleasure-enhancing biomedical and pharmaceutical solutions also lagging. The Pleasure Revolution is about understanding the many ways that sex happens, it is about consent and what it takes to have fulfilling sexual experiences. The unshackling of women's bodies, sexual desires and pleasure is the revolution for many women across the world and we need to be bold in reclaiming our sexual pleasure and sexual expression.

The last section of the book, Sexual Rights, contains important elements that must be respected and protected. I share my perspectives and show how in some aspects, as a society, we seem progressive yet when it comes to those who do not fit the mould, be it in their gender or sexual identity or in occupations such as sex work, we ourselves can be contributing to an unjust and unequal society.

I've included references to my work and experiences that some people may recognise from an article, a radio show or a television interview. As much as I have shared those details with you, I have brought all of myself to this book and had a wonderful journey going down memory lane to revisit my own experiences.

When women are able to hold conversations and negotiate the type of sex they want, including the use of condoms, toys and fantasy play, within respectful exchanges, the chances of good and affirming sexual experiences are greater. It is my wish that you find *A Guide to Sexual Health and Pleasure* informative and that you keep it as a reference tool that you keep going back to and it can assist in getting the best out of your consultation when you are face-to-face with your healthcare provider.

Enjoy!

Note for readers

I decided to use 'she' and 'women' but I am talking to all of you and the book is all inclusive! So that includes 'him', 'men', 'people', etc., etc.

I have included a few helpful (unfortunately not juicy as this isn't THAT kind of book!) pics and graphics to give you a bit more to think about and to orientate yourself.

I have sounded out some of the tricky anatomical words for you in the Sexual Health section. Not in a proper 'phonetic' kind of way, more of a 'as-you-hear-it' kind of way.

Look out for the 'Tips' that pop up every now and again. Denoted by 👍

Go to the back of the book for names, places and links to various medical and social services if you need advice and help. That's what they are there for!

Section 1

Sexual Health

Physiology

···

Vagina, vagina, vagina!

When last did you look at your vagina? Occasional stolen eye contact while grooming or bathing doesn't count. When last, if ever, did you take a mirror and just look? Okay, indulge me for a few moments. Put the book down, get into a comfortable position and take a good look. (Pro tip: ☺) selfie mode on your phone camera works just as well as a mirror!) I mean really look at it, the detail of the labia, the different openings on the vulva and get familiar with what your normal is.

Maybe you blushed or laughed so much that the tears made it hard for you to focus or maybe you only managed to stare at the pubic hair, but one thing is for certain we all have very different relationships with our vaginas and for as many reasons too. Self-examination of the genitals is seldom, if ever, spoken about or encouraged yet you are the perfect person to notice any changes and then seek advice. The path to learning, being comfortable, celebrating, and even reclaiming our bodies starts with the language we use to refer to our bodies, unlearning habits that do not serve us and relearning affirming ways of being sexual; looking, touching, feeling and exploring of your own bodies, emotions and expression.

I often wonder when the vulva, which encompasses the entire external parts of the genitalia, evolved to being referred to as 'the vagina'. Often what is referred to as 'the vagina' is in fact more accurately, the vaginal opening. Both in general discourse and in medical discussions, the details of the magnificence of that is the vulva has been reduced only to the mechanics of the vagina through which sometimes a foetus is birthed and many other times is feasted upon. The importance of naming body parts accurately and referring to them by their anatomical names cannot be overstated and continued lack of accuracy when referring to 'the vulva' is a form of erasure that is reductionist.

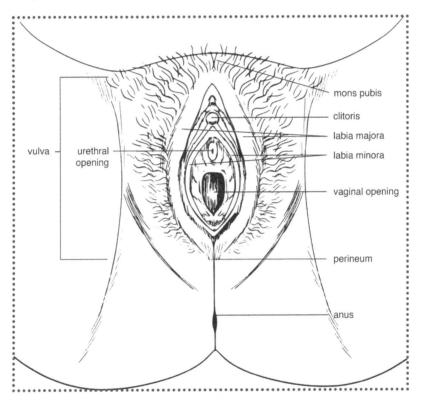

The vulva

Whenever I am asked to give 'the' sex talk, and I have done so to so many audiences, ranging from high school students in Orlando West, college students at West Virginia's Wesleyan College, during a session at a women's only conference entitled 'Let's talk about sex' in New Orleans and my favourite, healthy sex parties I host, one of my best icebreakers is to ask participants to say the 'name' of the vagina in their

Tip 👍 About your vulva

1. Quote me on this one: 'Your vagina is a self-cleansing machine' meaning that there is no need to use soaps or detergents.

2. Ingrown hair causes bumps on the skin around the groin and pubic areas. Exfoliating and applying moisturiser also helps to prevent build-up of dry skin if you are shaving or waxing your pubic area.

3. G-strings can predispose you to burning urine or thrush as the string can deposit faecal matter near the urethra and vaginal opening.

4. Be aware that your discharge will vary in colour, consistency and smell at different times throughout your menstrual cycle.

mother tongue. These words immediately, as I'm sure you can guess, make most people uncomfortable. I always ask that we say the words out loud and over and over again, enough times until the words start to sound less 'vulgar' (as many people say they are) and until, in fact, the reluctance to say the word out loud melts away.

Why and when did our anatomical parts become vulgar? How do we reclaim the use of language? Can we get to a point where in Sesotho or isiXhosa women can speak about their genitals without offence given or taken based on the experience of how such words are used and weaponised against us? There are so many words for 'vagina', in all languages, yet even as adults when we say any of these words out loud it's as if we are sharing a disapproving voice in our heads, be it of a parent, a caregiver, or a teacher. There is an expectation of and (often) a predictable backlash every time the word 'vagina' is said out loud.

Some adults never break the habit of referring to their own vaginas as food, inanimate objects, fluffy animals, flowers and others make up new words altogether, perhaps in an attempt to be less offensive. But is this really what is best? I don't think it is. By exceptionalising genitals and avoiding naming them correctly, it sends a message to children that there is something shameful about their private parts. In some cases, parents exhibit hysteria and even embarrassment when their kids do name their genitals as anatomically correct and sometimes even threaten punishment. Again this sends the wrong message to children; that there is something odd or unwelcome, dirty or wrong about their bodies. It is not possible to expect children to ignore or have no interest in their genitals. They do not share adults' cognitive processing or understand why they are being chastised or reprimanded. Because of adults' learnt behaviour, past experiences and reactions, it is not conducive to have affirming conversations with children. There is a large spectrum between normal inquisitiveness and children showing or interacting in inappropriate ways regarding language and behaviour around their bodies. The reaction to even what adults may consider inappropriate should still be informed.

On the other end of this spectrum, where the physical and sexual abuse of children is being handled by the justice system and children's courts, it is imperative that children are able to explain their body parts as accurately as possible during statement taking or cross-examination.

In the medical world, genitalia are discussed through a mechanical lens of conception, menstruation and urological function. There is very limited information at undergraduate or postgraduate level for doctors and nurses that deals with aspects of pleasure in a way that affirms sexual pleasure as part of health and wellness. The focus of disease processes and the resultant capitalistic commodification of sex, vaginal health and, by extension, general medicine through a pathological lens, means that the focus of sex through genitals and disease management has given rise to a pharmaceutical industry filled with 'alternative agents' claiming to be able to help women make themselves 'normal and healthy'. As if the vagina is by default in an abnormal state and needs to be improved. This trend is escalating and is evident in the number of harmful DIY treatments women are performing on their vulval area and vagina. Once, while on the radio open line, during a sexual health feature, a caller detailed how she had been inserting and washing her vagina with Epsom salts because she had heard it was good for the vagina. As a result, she had been experiencing what she described as a 'creamy discharge' intermittently throughout her cycle. By the end of the hour, many women had shared truly horrific stories of using concoctions such as snuff, fresh garlic and the dreaded over-the-counter feminine hygiene products.

Women everywhere are constantly discussing ways of making improvements to their vaginas; whether it be in online forums, in consultations with medics, in advertisements or with each other. Firstly, as I have said, it's a vulva and secondly, no two, three or four vulvas are the same and there is no standard shape or size of what is a 'good' or a 'bad' vulva. Every woman needs to know and accept her 'normal'.

So, let's get back to basics and look at what is actually 'down there'. The anatomical structure of the female genitalia is made up of the external genitals, comprising of the clitoris, labia minora, urethral opening, vaginal opening, and the inner genital tract consisting of the vaginal canal, G-spot, cervix, pelvic muscles, blood vessels, sweat glands and nerves.

If we start on the outside and look at what we can actually see, the pubic mound is made of fatty tissue and is called the mons pubis. Pubic hair (which is coming back into fashion apparently ☺) covers the mons pubis and that provides cushioning to the vulva and the fatty pad protects the pubic bone from trauma. If we move down towards the vaginal opening, the mons pubis splits into two 'lips' called the labia majora. These 'big lips' are (often) also covered in pubic hair and cover the smaller labia minora often referred to as the 'inner lips'. These mostly hairless folds of skin envelop the vaginal and urethral openings. Underneath the hood of the labia minora, at its top end, lies erectile tissue famously known as the clitoris. (Shame, there's so much yet to be written and told about the clitoris ☺.) I once received a tweet that read 'What would you ask on the first date' and I replied 'What is the clitoris'! As you can imagine, the responses went from mild to moderate to tremendously funny. But I digress; more on the clitoris later. ☺

As you move down, there is a smooth area with the urethra and the vaginal opening. The vaginal opening is right below your urethral opening. And then where the labia minora and majora join, is what is called the fourchette ('four-shet') and during childbirth, this is the tissue that is cut to enlarge the vaginal opening for a procedure called an episiotomy ('eh-pees-i-ot-omi').

There are various glands that function to provide lubrication to the genitals and the secretions lubricate the external genitalia during sexual arousal. These secretions are alkaline. The vaginal secretions have an acidic pH to prevent the growth of bacteria and yeast but this means that the vagina is an unfriendly environment for sperm. Sperm would therefore not make it past the vaginal canal due to the acidity and would be terminated, so an alkaline seminal fluid is produced to neutralise the acid and improve the survival of the sperm.

Internally, the vagina is an elastic tube and a muscular canal that connects the uterus, through the cervix that protrudes into the vagina. The lining of this 'canal' is ridged and this gives the vagina its textured feel.

Deep in the vagina is a layer of connective tissue with many elastin fibres that allow the vagina to stretch. A layer of smooth muscle tissue located even deeper allows the vagina to expand and contract. As a result, the vagina is very elastic and by design can stretch to accommodate a variety of things inserted into it, such as fingers, penises, sex toys, tampons and menstrual cups. During sexual penetration, the vagina is able to stretch in both length and diameter. During childbirth, the vagina acts as the 'passageway' for the baby; its elasticity allows it to greatly increase its diameter to accommodate the foetus. The vagina also provides a canal through which menstrual blood flows from the uterus, through the cervix and exits the body during menstruation.

16

If we go back to basic anatomy, the hymen is a thin membrane of tissue that surrounds and narrows the vaginal opening. This is the membrane that often tears or is broken during sexual intercourse. The anxieties and stress that many young women have about this tiny membrane and the pressure of some families placed on women to prove purity and virginity is immense. In my opinion, the hymen is the most overrated piece of anatomy. It saddens me that I talk to so many women who are anxious about maintaining and later proving their 'purity'. Some people are born with a very thin membrane that may be torn or ruptured by partaking in exercise such as horse riding and so may perforate or tear well before any sexual penetration, and may or may not leave a blood stain as evidence. It's therefore not an indication of being a virgin and the pressure to 'save it' for marriage is unnecessary and inaccurate.

Next comes the cervix, which is the structure that protrudes into the vagina and is part of the uterus (commonly referred to as the womb). The uterus has an estimated length of 5 to 7 centimetres and a width of 5 centimetres. It is 2.5 centimetres deep in its widest part (which I'm certain is much smaller than you thought, right?! ☺ and provides a place for implantation and growth for the foetus. The cervix can usually be felt at the end of your vagina if you insert your fingers deep enough. The cervix is a landmark that separates the vagina from the uterus and it is especially important to note that the uterus is a closed chamber so objects like sex toys or tampons cannot get 'lost' in there. Contrary to the myths that exist.

There is a tiny opening on the cervix that connects the uterus and vagina and it is through this opening that menstrual blood exits and where sperm can enter the uterus. The uterus is lined by the endometrium, which sheds every menstrual cycle to lead to menstrual blood flow.

The cervix, under certain circumstances, is able to stretch. When a procedure such as the insertion of an intrauterine device (IUD) or a tube called a cannula during manual vacuum aspiration (MVA) is performed, certain medication can be used to soften the cervix and help in the execution of these procedures. During childbirth this process is called dilation and is measured in centimetres. Once the cervix is fully dilated (to 10 centimetres) it allows for the passage of the foetus's head and body. The cervix is also the area that is sampled during a pap smear and during a vaginal examination and if there is an infection or inflammation present, the cervix might also be tender when palpated.

The uterus, a.k.a. the womb, is divided into three parts: the muscular body which is the main bulky looking part, the cervix at the bottom and the two fallopian tubes on either side. The uterus is lined by the thin endometrium ('en-dough-mee-tree-um'), which sheds every menstrual cycle and leads to menstrual blood flow. This monthly shedding is under the influence of hormones and should implantation occur, as a result of the ovum from the fallopian tube and sperm meeting, the growing embryo implants itself onto the endometrium which then provides support to the embryo during early development.

The deeper layers of the uterus are muscular and are important at birth as they contract to push the foetus through the birth canal. The fallopian tubes are a pair of tubes that extend from the left and right top corners of the uterus to the edge of the ovaries. The fallopian tubes also have muscle and at the ends have finger-like projections, the fimbriae, which move around the ovaries and catch a released egg, called the ovum, to carry them into the tube in order for them to reach the uterus. They are a passageway for the egg cells towards the uterus. The fallopian tube has a muscular layer that is responsible for the peristaltic movements that propel the ovum forward into the uterus.

Conception and implantation can occur within the tube, leading to ectopic pregnancy. The tubes are susceptible to infection that might damage their structures. Salpingitis, the inflammation of the fallopian tubes, is almost always caused by bacterial infections such as gonorrhoea, chlamydia and staphylococcus. The inflammation can result in excess fluid being produced around the affected tube and may cause adherence of the tube onto the intestines and as it heals, the scarring and blockage of the fallopian tubes make it difficult for sperm to travel through the tubes to get to the egg. This is still one of the most common causes of infertility. Whether the tube is damaged by infection, salpingitis, an ectopic pregnancy or endometriosis it is still possible to fall pregnant with the other functioning fallopian tube.

Conditions such as endometriosis or an ectopic pregnancy can result in surgery having to be performed on the tubes and may also lead to unfavourable changes in one or both of the tubes. The resultant scarring can also interfere with the ability of the tubes to carry the ova to the uterus. Every month, either the left or the right ovary releases an egg and it is therefore only one tube that is responsible, in that particular menstrual cycle, to deliver the egg to the uterus.

The ovaries are actually small glands located on the left and right sides of the uterus, near the fallopian tubes. Each ovary is shaped like an almond. The function of the ovary is to produce sex hormones – oestrogen ('es-truh-juhn') and progesterone – that are important in the maintenance of the secondary sex characteristics.

The cells that produce the ova, the eggs, are present from birth and reach maturity after puberty. Each month during ovulation, it is the mature ovum that is released. The ovum travels from the ovary to the fallopian tube, where it may be fertilised before reaching the uterus.

Let me tell you about the C.L.I.T.O.R.I.S

Now, let's talk about the clitoris. The clitoris is described in medical literature but is not always researched as well as other parts of the body and so its descriptions, function, role and purpose often lack the detail needed. Being the only organ in the human body whose sole purpose is for pleasure, and its only function is erogenous, the clitoris is somehow relegated to the not-so-important list of neuro-vascular anatomy to teach or learn. Yet the clitoris is one of the most magnificent parts of a woman's body, literally, with some of the best descriptions of it made as far back as 1844. An article in the *Journal of Urology* that studied the clitoral anatomy using micro-dissection, magnetic resonance imaging and three-dimensional reconstruction to provide some of the most comprehensive and accurate descriptions.

Most of the components of the clitoris are buried under the skin and connective tissue of the vulva. It is made up of a glans and hood, the only external components, and internally the part that is the most recognisable and often referred to as 'the bean', as well as other internal components. The clitoris is approximately 9 to 11 centimetres in size and its erogenous function is made possible by the network of nerves, together with erectile tissue and extensive blood supply, making the clitoris the centre for orgasmic response.

When a woman becomes aroused, the blood vessels become engorged and due to both pressure and touch sensitivity of the nerves, stimulation can result in pleasure not limited to the local area being stimulated, but the nerves transmit the sensation through the entire organ often leading to vaginal lubrication, pleasure and orgasm without penetration.

It is important to remember that your sexual well-being and pleasure is linked to your emotional, psychological and physical health. There are common medical conditions such as diabetes, hypertension and menopause and side-effects from various types of medication that can affect your ability to become aroused, have adequate lubrication and ultimately experience an orgasm.

Keep it tidy

Vaginas come in all shapes, sizes and colours and there is no one way for a vagina to look. For many years, genital piercings were the only common genital modification but recently there has been a surge in surgical and non-surgical interventions and many types of vaginal modifications. The popular areas for modification include the labia and vaginal walls, the inner thighs and the pubic area. Many people with concerns around the vaginal aesthetics are often already engaging in practices to alter either the smell or look of the vulva or the taste of vaginal fluids. The idea is to modify the vagina to meet the artificial standards set by society through narrow definitions and standards to achieve the 'designer vagina'.

Some of these modifications include vaginal bleaching, done mostly with creams to make the naturally darker skin tone of the vagina lighter, and vaginal contouring a.k.a. 'vontouring', a non-invasive non-surgical rejuvenation of the vaginal muscles and labia. Labioplasty, the most popular cosmetic surgery, is a procedure where the labia are reduced in size and made symmetrical. A 'vajazzle' is the adornment of the pubic area with decorations such as piercings, gemstones, crystals and glitter. Most recently, glitter balls or 'passion dust' are inserted into the vagina, where they dissolve and are supposed to add flavour and glitter to vaginal fluids. This 'glitter' can migrate into the uterus and even the fallopian tubes thereby causing various infections.

Many products meant for sexual enhancements are edible which means there is likely sugar in them that can lead to pH imbalances and the development of candida. It is not advisable to insert any products not tested for safety as the risk of sexually transmitted infections is far more likely.

There are many products available that promise great results but you need to look at the ingredients that make up these extracts, tinctures and mixtures, even on so-called natural remedies, prior to using these on the delicate tissue of the vagina.

Vaginal steaming is another fashionable grooming trend that is often described as a 'facial' for the vagina where a person sits over a bowl of steaming water often infused with various herbs in combination; rosemary for its antiseptic properties, marigold for wound healing and lemon balm to soothe cramps. There is no scientific evidence to support the need or use of vaginal steaming. It was first made fashionable and trendy when actress Gwyneth Paltrow espoused its benefits in the media. This procedure has been used in ancient medicine for centuries all over the world but the popularity of vaginal steaming has been seen in spas over the last decade and it has become popular as a cleanser for

> **What exactly is a douche?**
> A douche is something used to supposedly 'clean' the vaginal canal.
> Whether it's a spray, drops, a liner, wet wipes or a foam, all these devices
> are a detergent of some sort and will contain soap and will foam. But
> the vaginal canal doesn't need 'cleaning'; it's a self-cleansing machine. It
> cleanses itself in terms of the bacteria, the lactobacillus that grows there.
> NOTE: nothing needs to be inserted into the vagina to 'clean it' and that
> includes Savlon on a facecloth!
> BUT. The vulva needs cleaning. The vulva includes the groin, pubic hair,
> labia majora, labia minor etc and there are various bacteria that can grow
> as a result of sweating, etc., that need to be cleaned. Just remember
> there is a difference between a vagina and a vulva even though that's
> never mentioned when these so-called feminine products are being
> advertised.

the reproductive organs, including the uterus, cervix, and vagina.

The problem with this is that the vagina doesn't require 'cleaning' or 'cleansing'. The vaginal canal has a particular mixture of balanced normal flora called lactobacilli, and vaginal cleansing or steaming can alter this normal balance and may actually increase your risk of vaginal candidiasis. Practices such as douching have also been promoted in the past for vaginal cleansing but these are practices I strongly recommend you avoid.

There are medical conditions that can alter the appearance of the external genitalia, such as inflammation of the clitoris, genital ulcers on the vulva or perineum due to sexually transmitted infections, and vaginitis, which is a change in the normal balance of vaginal yeast and bacteria that can cause inflammation and redness around the vagina. Menopause can cause thinning of pubic hair. Vaginal dryness is a normal occurrence at different times during the menstrual cycle and can also result from a number of other factors or causes, such as breastfeeding, radiation or chemotherapy treatment for cancer, the surgical removal of the ovaries and some medications used to treat uterine fibroids or endometriosis, allergies and cold medications.

Certain antidepressants, douching and not enough foreplay before sex can all contribute to vaginal dryness. Childbirth and pregnancy also affect not only the level of lubrication in the vagina but also the appearance of the genitals.

Don't panic! It might just be an ingrown hair!

I receive so many frantic calls from women enquiring about the bumps and lumps they have discovered or felt on their mons pubis. Often these calls to the clinic are accompanied by so much anxiety and it is always interesting to hear the relief in a woman's voice once a diagnosis of a simple ingrown hair is made. Many women think anything 'abnormal' that appears around their genital area is a symptom of a sexually transmitted infection, whereas there are many dermatological disorders that can occur in the genital area, including the very common inflammation of the hair follicles as a result of ingrown hair. Ingrown hairs can affect anyone who shaves or waxes their pubic hair. This is usually self-limiting, meaning that one does not need antibiotics and the resolution is uneventful. Ingrown hair mostly occurs around the groin and pubic area in women (as well as in the armpits and on the legs) and, in men, on the chin, cheeks and around the beard area. Hair structure and direction of growth play a role in ingrown hairs. A curved hair follicle, which produces tightly curled hair, can cause the hair to re-enter the skin and grow sideways under the skin, rather than upward and outward. You might be prone to ingrown hair if you shave as shaving causes the hair to have sharp edges, especially if the skin is dry when shaved or pulled taut, as this allows the shaved hair to draw back into the skin and re-enter the skin without first growing out. Tweezing can also leave a hair fragment under the skin surface. Ingrown hairs can be itchy and uncomfortable and you may notice small, solid, rounded bumps called papules or pus-filled lesions called pustules. The embedded hairs might also be visible under the skin. There might be bacterial skin infection, hyper-pigmentation and scarring if the lesions become chronic. Mild infections caused by scratching the affected area may require an antibiotic ointment or oral antibiotics for more severe infection. A retinoid cream and an anti-inflammatory cream to reduce dead skin cells and inflammation may be prescribed.

Tip 👍
Avoid shaving, tweezing and waxing, if possible, while you have infected ingrown hair. Exfoliating and applying moisturiser also helps prevent the build-up of dry skin.

Intersex

Male and female sex organs develop from the same tissue. The chromosomes and the presence or absence of male hormones determines whether the male organs or female organs develop. In a foetus without a Y chromosome, therefore without the effects of male hormones, the developing genitals will mature as female. At birth, when the genitals do not clearly fit the physical appearance of what is expected to be male or female, they are said to be ambiguous. The genitals may not be fully developed or they may have characteristics of both male and female. The ambiguity may form part of other syndromes and genetic conditions or it may occur as a single characteristic. There are many variations and the penis may be very small or not visible at all, with the presence of some testicular tissue. In some cases there may be both testicular and ovarian tissue present inside the pelvis.

The term 'intersex' is thrown around a lot these days but the 'actual' definition refers to people who are born with genetic, hormonal or physical sex characteristics that do not fit the medical definitions of exclusively male or female. It does not, by the way, determine sexual orientation or gender identity. We are all assigned a gender at birth, based on how our external genitalia look, either female or male. Intersex children have genital characteristics that represent a minority in terms of the general population and this pressure to assign sex in the binary of female or male informs the pressure experienced by caregivers and healthcare providers.

The many variations in characteristics of external and internal genitalia, such as length, girth, skin tone, appearance and ability to carry a pregnancy, are not the sole determinants of gender, of ability to have sexual pleasure or predictors of sexual health. Intersex people often face a significant amount of bullying and pressure to commit to unwanted, often ill-timed, medical procedures and medications, as a way to attempt to correct how people are naturally born in order to wrongfully force the way sexual and reproductive anatomy fit in narrow definitions of what is female or male. Their families also experience discrimination and abuse and violence because they often have a deeper outlook on the diversity of bodies and gender.

Those who are genetically female (with two X chromosomes) could present with a clitoris that is large and may resemble a penis. The labia may have folds resembling a scrotum and may be closed. There may also be lumps that, when palpated, are like testes in the labia that have fused.

Those who are genetically male (with one X and one Y chromosome) may have a small penis, with the urethra not fully extending to the tip of the penis and the penis may have the urethral opening closer to the scrotum. There could also be an absence of one or both testicles and the area that appears to be the scrotum. When one or both testes remain in the lower abdominal cavity, the condition is called undescended testes. The scrotum may resemble labia. Undescended testes is a common medical condition and may occur on its own, without being part of a genetic syndrome. The consensus is that 1.7% of the global population has intersex traits, which means one to two babies in every one hundred born. This estimate was published in the *American Journal of Human Biology* and is the most accurate estimate we currently have in the medical world.

When a child is born intersex, the doctors and the family decide on a gender and raise the baby as that gender. Legally, intersex is not recognised and people are forced to identify as either male or female. Section 2 of the Constitution gives intersex people the right to define a gender identity, but on the birth certificate, the biological sex is still female or male. It is common for so-called surgical correction to be performed on the newborn or toddler's genitals and in some cases the person is given male or female hormones around puberty. The concerns about the child's future fertility depend on the specific diagnosis. Some disorders of sex development are associated with an increased risk of certain types of cancer. Awareness of intersex is slowly growing but much, much more needs to be done.

Penis, penis, penis!

The typical male genitalia and reproductive system are located inside and outside of the pelvis. They include the penis and the testicles located outside of the pelvis. The penis is an organ that has a urinary function as well as a sexual function and the growth and size of the penis reaches its mature size during puberty. There are several parts to the penis, namely the head of the penis called the glans, the foreskin called the prepuce that covers the glans and, if circumcised, this soft lining on the head becomes dry skin. The urinary pipe, called the urethra runs through the penis to allow for the passage of urine out of the body. Sperm also passes through the urethra.

In order to have erectile abilities, the penis has columns of sponge-like tissue along the sides and it is this tissue that leads to an erection when it is filled with blood. The vas deferens, which is a Latin phrase meaning 'carrying-away vessel', is a muscular tube that carries sperm to the outside of the body, during ejaculation. The epididymis ('eh-pee-dih-dih-mis') is a coiled tube that helps with the maturation of sperm. During ejaculation the contractions transport the sperm to the vas deferens. The testicles are oval in shape and produce sperm and

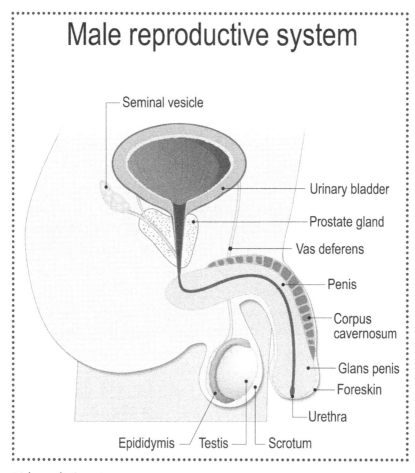

Male reproductive system

Seminal vesicle

Urinary bladder

Prostate gland

Vas deferens

Penis

Corpus cavernosum

Glans penis

Foreskin

Urethra

Epididymis   Testis   Scrotum

Male reproductive system

testosterone. The testicles hang outside the pelvis in what is called the scrotum. The skin of the scrotum helps regulate the temperature of the testicles. This is important because sperm requires a cooler body temperature for development. Pre-ejaculation fluid may contain sperm and the amount of fluid released can be up to 4 millilitres, which means a woman can fall pregnant even when full ejaculation doesn't occur inside the vagina. Although the actual number of sperm in the pre-ejaculation fluid is lower, the concentration and motility of sperm is equivalent to ejaculate, hence why the chances of pregnancy remain. It is not possible to keep pre-ejaculation or ejaculation away from the vulva or entering the vagina every time you have sex. Withdrawal of the penis from the vagina before ejaculation is unreliable at best and offers no protection from sexually transmitted infections. Statistically, every year, about 22 out of 100 women who use the withdrawal method fall pregnant. That's about 1 in 5.

Ejaculated sperm remain viable for several days within the female reproductive tract and fertilisation can occur for as long as the sperm remain alive. This can be as much as five days. Every time ejaculation happens, the semen can contain up to 500 million sperm. Once deposited into the vagina, the sperm, aided by contractions of the uterus, travel through the cervix and into the uterus. If a mature ovum is in one of the fallopian tubes, one of the sperm can penetrate it and at that stage fertilisation happens.

Some common sexual health-related conditions can be anatomical, some physiological and others a result of complications of other chronic illnesses, medication or injury. Erectile dysfunction, for example, is where the penis does not reach the level of hardness for satisfying penetration. Hypospadias ('hy-po-spay-di-as') is a birth defect in which the urethra is at the bottom or top of the head of the penis and not at the tip. It is not all that uncommon and in most cases surgery can correct hypospadias. A hydrocele ('hydro-seal') is a condition where fluid collects in the membranes surrounding the testes. The swollen scrotum is a common sign and surgery may be indicated. Phimosis ('fee-mo-sis') and paraphimosis ('para-fee-mo-sis') are conditions where the foreskin cannot be retracted or if retracted cannot be returned to its normal position over the penis head, requiring surgery to correct. Inflammation of the glans of the penis, can involve the foreskin of an uncircumcised penis, which can lead to pain, tenderness and redness of the penis head and sometimes requires antibiotic treatment. Sometimes the curvature at the end of the penis and shaft may be abnormal and may be present at birth. In adults, injury can cause abnormalities in shape and, if severe, may be corrected by surgery.

Circumcision

The health benefits of circumcision are often discussed and the relationship between sensitivity post the circumcision remains a common question. Some of the benefits of circumcision include a decreased risk of urinary tract infections and less risk of acquisition of some sexually transmitted diseases. Circumcision also makes it easier to keep the end of the penis clean. If a man is not circumcised, it is important to clean the foreskin specifically, by gently pulling the foreskin backwards, cleaning the skin underneath with soap and water and then pulling the foreskin forwards again. This should be done every day to avoid a build-up of dirt under the foreskin.

The hormonal orchestra: Puberty

The stages of puberty follow a predictable sequence, although some people may undergo puberty earlier than others. People usually start going through puberty between the ages of eight and 14. During puberty, the body undergoes many changes both physical and emotional. Those with female characteristics and hormonal influences often start puberty before those with male characteristics. Puberty develops in stages and takes several years to complete. Our bodies are unique and therefore some people may experience certain changes earlier and others later; puberty is different for each person.

For those with male characteristics, an Adam's apple (bump in your throat) may develop and become visible. You might experience a lower or deeper voice that can crack while it's changing. The penis and testicles get bigger. The growth of hair on the face, chest and back may be dramatic.

For those with female characteristics, there may be swelling around the nipples and some breast tissue may grow. The hips get wider, the shoulders may get broader. The labia may change in colour and size and the hormonal influences in those with ovaries and a uterus may lead to the first menstrual period.

Although normal, puberty can come with heightened and intense anxiety, excitement and some confusion. I know that what seemed like informal chats with my mother about her body and what changes my body would undergo, went a long way in making me feel less weird and I was not stressed by the changes. It was helpful to have her share some of her experiences and I looked forward to puberty because of my mom. I had an idea of what to expect in terms of bodily changes and it was only much later on in high school that I realised most girls were not particularly looking forward to menstruation and that my excitement and anticipation was uncommon.

Menstrual Health

My first period

It was November 2016 and I woke up and realised that the dull ache in my lower back was the usual period pain and although I had an adequate supply of tampons, I just couldn't bear the thought of shoving another tampon in my vagina. I think the word 'shove' explains this monthly process well, as I had grown to dread it more and more. Pads weren't an option as I had last used them after giving birth and found them very uncomfortable. I also remember how I had to use up to three pads at a time in high school during sports activities and how horrified I was at the thought of leaking while playing sport. Imagine what a maxi tampon plus three layered pads felt like, while kitted in goalie kit, during a game of hockey.

My relationship with my menstruation was not always filled with dread and discomfort. Even today, with all the pain and premenstrual changes affecting me, I still have an overall positive experience of my body and my relationship with my cycle.

The current global and national focus on menstrual hygiene has brought with it discussions around the accessibility and affordability of options presented to young women. However, these campaigns need to be more inclusive and offer young women more than pads or tampons as solutions. We need to approach the issue with a broader understanding of the life cycle of a tampon, pad, menstrual cup or reusable pad and what all these different options mean for environmental health. Why

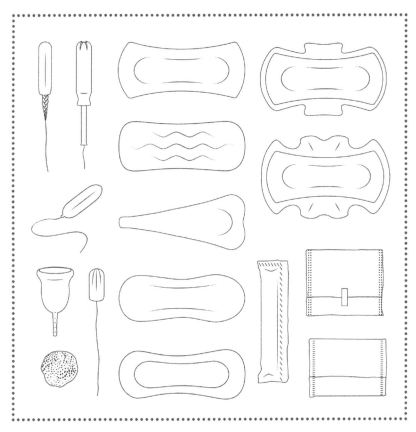

Feminine hygiene products

did tampons and pads become the only solution for women the world over? And why, even in places where there are other menstrual products, do we still limit our choice to pads and tampons?

One hot summer's day, 12-year-old me had had a somewhat uneventful day at school and when I arrived home I immediately went to the bathroom. I was in the habit of looking at the toilet paper I used to wipe myself after weeing because I had been eagerly anticipating the arrival of my period. I don't recall the exact words my mother used but I remember the main details were that a period was something wonderful to celebrate and it meant I had become a woman.

When I saw red that day on the piece of toilet paper, I screamed at the top of my voice. I didn't even flush the toilet before I ran to the phone in my mom's bedroom to call her at work. She ran her own supermarket about 20 kilometres away from our house in a village called Tsheseng in Qwaqwa. She answered the phone and I yelled, 'Hahahaha ke ngwanana jwale, I have my periods at last.' I told her to come home right away and that I'd keep the tissue for her. She reminded me where we kept the pad collection in preparation for this day, in an attempt to calm me down, but there was no way I'd forgotten!

Thereafter, every month after my period started, my mom and I would bond over which pads were best and what combination of pain medication worked best for my cramps. I remember going to our family doctor and I recall him discussing my sprouting breasts, growing hips and what all the changes to my body meant.

Menstruation typically begins at approximately the age of 12, but it has been documented that menstrual periods are possible as early as age eight. Given this timing, it is quite obvious that delaying sexuality and health discussions with girls until their early teens, is a bit late. Because of the association with blood, and I suppose for some young women it's scary to see blood that has come from the vagina, many parents and caregivers make the mistake of centring 'The Sex Talk' around this event and neglect to provide a comprehensive talk of all things sexual health-related.

The earlier you can begin talking to young people about the changes to expect during puberty, the better and more equipped they will be. I always advise parents and caregivers not to plan a single tell-all discussion. Sexuality and health education should happen from the moment we teach children about body parts. It should be in the series of conversations held throughout the years when children may ask questions about menstruation, body changes, feelings they have about their bodies, their fears and concerns. These conversations will provide an opportunity for caregivers to answer openly and honestly.

Some young people do not ask questions and will not actively seek you out for 'the talk' so it is up to you to start the conversation. Having a warm and inviting communication style means that it will be easier for children to approach you. If it is something you don't know, don't lie. Rather find out the answers and, if appropriate, look for the answers with the children doing the asking. It is not easy to have the required knowledge to pass on, especially if you are an adult who did not receive comprehensive sexuality education. It requires learning and confronting your own fears or prejudices that you may have towards sex, gender and sexual expression. The associated fear and embarrassment is real, especially when you are not confident, but the only way to get confident is to learn the language and details in order to be a trustworthy resource for young people.

You might start by asking what your child knows about puberty, sexuality and gender. Clarify any misinformation, use simple language and the language they are using in terms of slang and offer accurate anatomical terms where necessary. Explain the basics and share your own challenges and experiences; this will go a long way. You might need to follow up and find out from the teachers who are in charge of life orientation or sex education at school to gauge the level of engagement or difficulties the child might be having. This is not a single event, it requires interest in the child's holistic health and wellness.

What is the menstrual cup?

The menstrual cup has been garnering a lot of attention, especially since endorsements from the likes of the model Amber Rose and other celebrities, but the cup has always been around. Where possible, young women should be afforded an opportunity to learn about the cup and get the necessary demonstrations. This is needed due to the relative lack of knowledge available.

The cup can last from eight to 10 years. Because it is made of silicone, it warms up to body temperature and as a result of its shape, it moulds itself easily to the vaginal canal.

In every single talk I have delivered when discussing the cup, the issue

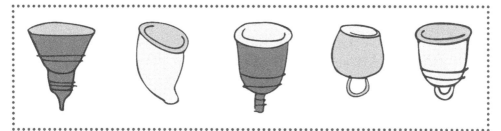

Menstrual cups

of virginity comes up. I use those moments to delve deeper into the questions about why women are burdened with maintaining purity and for whose benefit is the obsession with hymens. And is the concern and idea of 'breaking' our virginity working for women and our relationships with our vaginas and how we relate to sex and being sexual? To what extent are the teachings and missions about our bodies, the timing of bodily processes and aesthetics of the vagina, tied up to the idea that women are valued for how long they can maintain this so-called purity?

I decided to live-tweet my first experience trying the menstrual cup, so, yes, you really will find a thread on my timeline about manoeuvring a cup into the right place in your vagina! I was inquisitive about the insertion and feel of the cup and knew that many of my followers would be too. I had Googled a health shop nearby that stocked menstrual cups and purchased my first one. There was a fair selection in the shop so it wasn't difficult to find them once I was there.

When I got home, I got ready to fit the cup but while attempting to insert it, it slid out of my hands! Luckily I managed to grab it before it fell on the floor! I re-folded it and placed the cup inside my vagina but it didn't feel right so on the next attempt I decided to use warm water to soften the silicone. I folded the cup into a wrinkle in a shape of a U and inserted it a few centimetres into my vaginal canal. I followed the instructions on the leaflet to push it in as far as I could, heard a small pop and knew that I had got it right.

Even after the wobbly first attempts, I knew I had made the right decision in choosing the cup. It didn't feel any more uncomfortable than

35

using a tampon. I did wonder about the possibility of leaks and if I had actually placed it correctly so I gave it about an hour before I went to check. I thought I'd give the blood a chance to collect and I was pleasantly surprised – no spills, no mess.

I removed the cup, rinsed it in the basin and reinserted it. I felt confident so I decided to go out and walk around the mall. I went to the toilet to wee but didn't remove it and a few minutes later I felt a little uncomfortable. I realised that maybe I needed to push it in a bit further, which I did, and felt better immediately. Later in the day while using the public toilets, I wiped the cup dry with tissue as opposed to rinsing it. Overall it was a successful day and I felt good about the experience.

A few months later, I decided to buy a smaller size menstrual cup and the fit was even better. The menstrual cup has brought me so much closer to my periods as a whole; the experience of being a woman and my actual menstrual blood in terms of the colour, the smell and consistency. I'll never go back.

I understand how intimidating the thought of inserting the cup can be but relax, take a deep breath and give it a go! You'll thank me later!

Tip 👍
....

Sterilise your menstrual cup in the microwave or submerge it in a pot of boiling water and always use a silicone disinfectant spray. The same one you use to clean your sex toys. ☺

Toxic shock syndrome

Whenever the topic of menstruation is discussed, the issue of toxic shock syndrome always comes up when talking about tampons. This condition is rare but it is a life-threatening complication of certain types of bacterial infections: most commonly that of staphylococcus aureus (staph) bacteria.

Toxic shock syndrome was associated primarily with the use of the older super-absorbent-type tampons. However, since manufacturers removed certain types of tampons from the market, the incidence of toxic shock syndrome in menstruating women has declined over the years. The use of materials in tampons and pads that were associated with toxic shock syndrome is said to have declined and the Food and Drug Administration requires labelling for absorbency levels of tampons and for guidelines to be printed on boxes. The standard advice is to read the information on the packaging and change tampons frequently; at least every four to eight hours.

Toxic shock syndrome can affect anyone, not only women who are using tampons. Possible signs and symptoms of toxic shock syndrome include: a high fever, vomiting or diarrhoea, a rash on the palms and soles of the feet, muscle aches and headaches. About half the cases of toxic shock syndrome associated with staphylococcus bacteria occur in women of menstruating age; the rest occur in older women, men and children.

Other conditions such as cuts or burns on the skin, recent surgical procedures and viral infections have also been associated with toxic shock syndrome. Toxic shock syndrome can progress rapidly and can cause sepsis in severe cases.

PMS

Premenstrual syndrome (PMS), also known as 'premenstrual tension' (PMT), occurs in the days after ovulation, leading up to a menstrual period. About 90% of women experience premenstrual symptoms at some point in their lives. Many women experience PMS characterised by various physical and psychological symptoms that can start from a few days to two weeks before a menstrual period. The intensity of PMS can range from very mild to severe. Hormonal fluctuations after ovulation, certain sensitivity to the rising progesterone and decrease in oestrogen, chemical messengers in the brain, genetics and environmental factors can all affect the chances of experiencing PMS.

Most women experience milder forms of PMS characterised by breast tenderness, abdominal discomfort, bloating, headaches, lower back ache, joint and muscle aches. Water retention, poor sleep, skin break-outs and certain food cravings are also common. Some women have problems concentrating, mood swings, irritability and exhaustion that may lead to frustration.

Severe PMS can affect a woman's quality of life and her relationships, leading to a sense of a loss of control over one's body and emotions, as experienced by about 20% to 40% of all girls and women. This can be so severe that it significantly affects mental health in the form of anxiety or depression and is known as premenstrual dysphoric disorder (PMDD), which affects between 3% to 8% of women. Because of the prejudiced views that women are irrational and unpredictable at certain times of the month, many women have a hard time sharing their experiences of PMS and thus lose out on possible support from a partner, family and friends. Many women who experience PMS cannot take time off work to recover or seek medical care.

Managing the impact of PMS is one of the most stressful and anxiety-inducing situations for many women. The expected ridicule and constant teasing about very real physical and emotional symptoms makes it hard for some women to cope, thereby worsening their anxiety and frustration. PMS and its severity can vary from month to month and change over time. It is possible to track your symptoms and keep a diary that you can share with your doctor for a thorough consultation, and there is medication that can be prescribed to ease some of the symptoms of PMS.

Sexual desire also naturally changes and wanes throughout the menstrual cycle and the increase in desire for sex around ovulation is a known and recognised part of a normal cycle. This is not commonly spoken of outside of relationships women perceive as safe, partly because the sexual pleasure of women, often and unnecessarily, gets conflated with morality, sin and forbidden lust. Many women notice the difference or surge in their sexual desire but this does not always result in more sexual intercourse as some of the other symptoms that cause discomfort turn women off sex. The interplay and resulting fluctuations of all the hormones result in a hormonal orchestra and the desire for sexual activity and pleasure may last well into menstruation. Some women do not experience a surge in sexual desire and that too is normal.

Many communities in rural areas still hold the belief that menstruating women are dirty, that they will contaminate the home or anger the gods and as a result of this deep-seated belief, millions of young women are isolated from their families and sleep in huts or sheds that do not offer protection from extreme cold or heat. A 21-year-old woman died in Nepal in 2018 after suffering smoke inhalation while trying to keep warm in an area away from the rest of the community due to her being ostracised while having her period.

I attended an all-girls school but even in that environment, we didn't speak freely about our periods. We used 'code words' and hid our pads and tampons away. Who were we going to offend?! Why did

---

There are more than 5 000 different phrases/words/euphemistic expressions used to talk about and describe periods; proof of the stigma STILL surrounding menstruation. Why don't we call it by its name?!

Ever heard of these?!
Red robot, red Lamborghini (who knew, right?!☺), moon time, monthlies, on the rag, visit from Auntie Flo, crimson tide, riding the cotton pony, shark week, girl flu, checking into the red roof inn, Eve's curse, lady in red, monthly subscription, Raggedy Anne, the sacred dance of the uterus, taking Carrie to the prom, saving Ryan's privates, serving box wine, paper cut, the painters are in, on the blob, leak week, jam sandwich, the hunt for red October, flying the Japanese flag, bitch is back, bloody Mary, clean-up in aisle one, devil's juice, high tide, little Miss strawberry. You get the point!☺

Physical signs of PMS

Bloating

Abdominal cramps

Tenderness of the breasts and nipples

Noticeable increase in appetite

Headaches and worsening of migraines

Muscle aches

Swollen ankles

Worsening of pimples or a fresh breakout of new pimples

Most commonly diarrhoea, although some people experience constipation

Emotional signs

Depressed mood

Crying

Mood swings

Insomnia

Feeling overwhelmed

Anxiety

Behavioural signs

Fatigue

Poor memory

Poor concentration

we hide everything?! One thing is certain: even worlds apart, thousands of kilometres away, one thing women have in common is that the stigma around menstruation is deep. This is why the global movement aimed at normalising menstruation is vital. Whether it be dealing with a bloodstain on clothing without being judgemental, the buying of pads or tampons without feeling awkward or shameful, discussing menstruation in a positive light with young people and ensuring that healthcare providers manage the pain and other symptoms optimally, all these small acts matter in the bigger revolution of normalising menstruation.

Pain management

When I became a doctor I realised how many women were not being taken seriously when they complained of menstrual cramps and cycle irregularity and that many primary health facilities do not stock medicine required for an optimal, step-up approach to pain management. Many women suffer terribly during ovulation, in the days leading up to the menstrual period and during menstruation. For most, the option available is paracetamol taken on its own, and sometimes in combination with an anti-inflammatory such as Ibuprofen.

The gender bias, as well as racial medical bias that relegates black women's bodies to objects designed to endure pain, combined with sub-optimal pain management, reinforces the belief that there is a certain level of pain and suffering that womanhood comes with and that, in fact, periods were meant to be suffered through. This is not true. Many women are self-medicating using over-the-counter medication and do not receive optimal analgesic combinations suitable for them.

Consult your healthcare provider if your quality of life is negatively impacted by your menstruation, if you are unable to go to work or study due to one or more of the following issues:
- Your menstrual periods stop for more than 90 days and you are not pregnant
- Your periods become irregular or unpredictable after previously being regular
- You bleed for more than seven days and this is uncommon for you

- You bleed more heavily than usual or soak through more than one pad or tampon every two hours
- Your menstrual cycle is less than 21 days or more than 35 days apart
- You bleed between periods
- You develop severe uncommon pain during your period.

Heavy menstrual bleeding is very common with approximately one-third of women worldwide seeking treatment for it. The medical term for it is menorrhagia ('men-oh-rah-jee-uh'). There are several symptoms that may be present to indicate a woman might be suffering from menorrhagia:

- Bleeding lasts more than seven days
- Bleeding soaks through one or more tampons or pads every hour for several hours in a row
- Needing to wear more than one pad at a time to control menstrual flow
- Needing to change pads or tampons during the night
- Menstrual flow that contains blood clots that are large and recurring.

Possible causes of menorrhagia vary from hormonal, uterine, ovarian or other medical disorders, as well as side effects from certain medications. The most common medical causes include: polycystic ovary syndrome (PCOS), obesity, insulin resistance and thyroid problems. Cancer of the uterus or cervix is another cause and understanding your risk factors as well as screening tests remain most important for early cancer diagnosis. If you are pregnant, conditions such as a spontaneous miscarriage or ectopic pregnancy, can cause abnormal bleeding. Certain medications such as anti-thrombotic injections and tablets can also cause increased bleeding. Untreated heavy or prolonged bleeding that keeps you from doing the things you would do normally can have an ongoing impact on your quality of life and can also cause anaemia.

People have different perceptions of what 'heavy menstrual bleeding' is, so it is important to seek advice from your doctor or nurse who will ask you about your medical history and menstrual cycles and advise you on a way forward.

Some gynaecological conditions can be hereditary and your doctor may also ask if any of your family members have had heavy menstrual bleeding. You can expect to have a pelvic exam, an ultrasound, pap smear, blood tests and imaging investigations, where appropriate, when seeking advice about menstruation. The type of management will depend on the cause of your bleeding and medical, surgical and supportive therapies will be taken into consideration. The issue of comfort and optimal medical management is incomplete without ensuring dignity for those who are transgender and require advice and suitable hygiene products.

One of the reasons why annual gynaecological check-ups are recommended is to pick up any changes early and track the progression of certain conditions. Depending on the type of contraception method being used, for example, birth control pills and intrauterine devices (IUDs) or injectables, you may experience alteration in your menstrual cycle.

A quick anatomy lesson

The complete female reproductive cycle usually takes about 28 days on average, but may be as short as 24 days or as long as 36 days for some. The cycle is counted from the first day of the current period to the first day of the next period. The menstrual cycle is the normal cyclic shedding of the uterine lining, the endometrium, in response to the interactions of hormones. Midway through the cycle, between days 12 and 16, ovulation occurs. Interestingly, around ovulation, the quantity of vaginal discharge can increase 30-fold leading to breast tenderness, abdominal cramps and, in some people, premenstrual syndrome starts soon after this.

These increased vaginal secretions will be noticeable a week or so

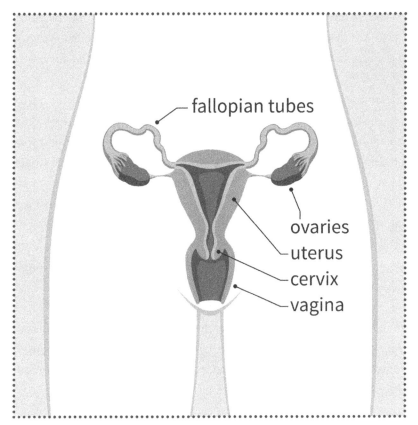

Female reproductive system

prior to your period. After ovulation, as progesterone levels rise, the cervical mucous becomes thick, viscous and opaque. The factors that affect the amount and consistency of the secretions are not limited to changes in hormonal levels of oestrogen and progesterone. See the box below for some of the factors to be aware of.

A drop in oestrogen levels reduces the amount of moisture available. During the follicular phase, the oestrogen levels rise as the new egg grows and matures. Oestrogen helps to maintain that lubricating fluid and keeps the lining of your vagina healthy, thick and elastic.

If the egg is not fertilised, levels of oestrogen and progesterone decrease and without the high levels of hormones to help maintain

Tip 👍
....

If you find the vaginal discharge is copious, has an odour or contains any blood, it is best to go for a medical check-up to ensure that you are not overlooking treatable medical causes. Discharge will vary in colour, consistency and odour at different times throughout your menstrual cycle.

PS While on the topic of 'smell', let's be clear that there is no 'natural' smell when it comes to genitals. Each person's body odour is influenced by hormonal changes, bacterial growth on the skin surrounding the area and the presence of pubic hair. Consult your doctor if you have an odour you are concerned about as many infections do alter the smell and type of discharge.

The following factors may have an effect on the vaginal wall lining and cervix:

Sexual excitement and arousal

Use of lubricants during intercourse

Vaginal infection or sexually transmitted disease

Douching

Pregnancy

Breastfeeding

Peri-menopause

Surgery or procedures performed on the cervix

it, the thick womb lining, the endometrium, that has built up starts to break down, and the body sheds the lining. This is the start of a period and the beginning of the menstrual cycle.

If fertilisation occurs, the menstrual cycle stops and the fertilised egg is called a zygote and contains 46 chromosomes. Half of the chromosomes, 23, are from the ovum and half of the genetic material is from the sperm. The zygote divides over and over, travels down the fallopian tubes and implants in the uterus. The uterus is the area where the growth and maturation of the zygote occurs; into an embryo, then a foetus and, finally, at birth, a baby.

Even if you have had sex during your most fertile time, there are many other factors that affect your ability to conceive. It can take healthy people more than 12 months to conceive and, typically, doctors will start investigating for infertility only after 12 months of regular sex when ovulation occurs.

Tip 👍
....

If you notice anything 'out of the ordinary' when it comes to any of the following factors, consult your healthcare professional:

- A change in colour, odour or amount of vaginal discharge
- Vulval redness, itching or irritation
- Vulval bleeding between periods, after sex or after menopause
- A mass or bulge in your vagina.

The days around ovulation are the most fertile time during your cycle and is when an egg is released from one of the ovaries. Ovulation tests are approximately 99% accurate in detecting the hormone surge that precedes ovulation. It can be difficult for some people, particularly if their cycles are irregular, to track ovulation so the use of ovulation urine tests are invaluable. In my personal experience, there are more women with mobile applications to track periods than not.

Of the 53 top websites and smartphone apps the research published in the *Journal of Obstetrics and Gynaecology* analysed, only four – one website and three apps – accurately predicted the most fertile window. This study revealed that most of these fertility trackers provide inaccurate fertile windows. Keeping an ovulation calendar based on counting days, using basal body temperature or saliva changes are less accurate than hormone monitoring and are more likely to be affected by other variables.

The best option is the urine ovulation test home kit. You can start keeping a record of your menstrual cycle on a calendar, diary or on a mobile app. You will need to start tracking the start and end date every month for a few months in order to establish a pattern and to identify the changes to your cycle. Keeping a period or menstrual diary can be of great value when you are consulting your healthcare provider.

Even if you are healthy and have no real reason to be concerned, it is still valuable to take note of the following details:

- Start date: the day of the first sight of blood
- End date: the last day of bleeding
- Flow: does the flow seem lighter or heavier than usual? How often do you need to change your sanitary pad, tampon or cup? Have you seen any blood clots? Are clots a new occurrence or common with your period?
- Abnormal bleeding: are you bleeding in-between periods? For how many days?
- Pain: describe any pain associated with your period. Has the pain evolved or is it worse than usual? Is it in the same area every month?
- Other changes: have you noted any significant change such as change in the colour of the blood?

Irregularities to the menstrual cycle can have many different causes. Some common causes include but are not limited to:

- Pregnancy – Although some people experience spotting during pregnancy, bleeding is considered abnormal and the lack of ovulation causes the halt to the menstrual cycle.

- Breastfeeding – Typically, the return of menstruation after pregnancy can be delayed by exclusive breastfeeding. It is, however, possible to ovulate and get pregnant while breastfeeding and as a result a contraceptive method ideal for breastfeeding is encouraged.
- Eating disorders such as anorexia nervosa, extreme weight loss or excessive exercising can disrupt menstruation.
- Polycystic ovary syndrome (PCOS) – Women with this common endocrine system disorder may have irregular periods.
- Premature ovarian failure – This refers to the loss of normal ovarian function before the age of 40. This is not menopause because it occurs at an early age. It can occur over a period of many years.
- Pelvic inflammatory disease (PID) – This infection of the internal reproductive organs can cause irregular menstrual bleeding.
- Uterine fibroids – These are growths of the smooth muscle of the uterus. Fibroids can cause heavy menstrual periods and prolonged menstrual periods.
- Endometriosis – A disorder in which the endometrium grows outside your uterus. This abnormal endometrial tissue continues to be reactive to hormones, causing pain and discomfort in the pelvic and abdominal areas.

Termination of pregnancy

Very few medical procedures are as much of a subject of morals and religion as the choice to terminate a pregnancy. The most important thing, putting differences aside, is that no person should die, live with complications or experience harassment and sub-optimal medical care due to an unwanted pregnancy. As medical providers, it is incumbent on us all to place the health and wellbeing of patients ahead of our personal feelings and as experts treat all patients with dignity. The same way we do not discriminate against patients who differ in standing in morals such as injured drunk drivers or prisoners in need of medical care, we should protect the rights of those who do not wish to be pregnant. The management of the termination of pregnancy is informed by research and protocols giving healthcare providers the clinical guidance.

One of the main reasons I could never quit social media, is the large number of people who enquire, on a daily basis, about access to safe abortion. I feel anxious when I think of how many people need information and wonder how many more there are, without access to social media or not aware of people like myself who have become a resource for those needing information.

Usually I get asked for the details of actual health facilities people can visit and it shocks me how many people still think that having an abortion is an illegal act.

The right to decide if you want children and if you do, how many you want and when to carry a pregnancy to full-term is a human right. The decision whether or not the timing of a pregnancy is suitable is personal and consent to stop a pregnancy from progressing remains that of the pregnant person. In some instances, the circumstances leading to a pregnancy may make the pregnancy and child-rearing unsupportable.

The reasons are many and varied and the patient profile is diverse. I have performed abortion procedures for married couples, single women, older women, people who have undergone assisted fertility treatment, young people, wealthy people, poor people, older women who are peri-menopausal, women who were on contraceptives and still experienced failure, and so many others. The bottom line is that the main reason people request a termination is because the pregnancy is unsupportable. None of these people should be burdened with victimhood or self-loathing in order for their circumstances to be deemed worthy.

The stigma and obstruction experienced by those who undergo the medical procedure and those health professionals who offer the

ABORTION: SOUTH AFRICA

Safe Abortion Access is a Human Right.

'We demand literal access to dignified, timeous, evidence-based care.'
DR TLALENG MOFOKENG (MBChB)

KNOW YOUR RIGHTS!

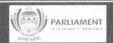

Bill of Rights:
Chapter 2, Section 27 sets out a number of rights with regard to health, including right to access to health care, including Reproductive Rights.

CHOICE ON TERMINATION OF PREGNANCY ACT 92 OF 1996

0-12 WEEKS

An abortion may be performed at the request of the woman (pregnant person)

13-20 WEEKS

If it endangers the woman's mental or physical health,
if the foetus may suffer from a severe mental or physical abnormality,
if pregnancy resulted from rape or incest or
if it would significantly affect the woman's social or economic circumstances.

21 WEEKS AND ABOVE

If it could endanger the woman's life,
if the foetus is severely malformed, or
if there is a risk of severe injury to the foetus.

termination is immense and is experienced regardless of age, marital status, class or race. In South Africa, the Bill of Rights in the Constitution guarantees and recognises access to healthcare, including reproductive health as a right.

In 1996, The Choice on Termination of Pregnancy (CTOP) Act was adopted and this Act provides the legal framework for the provision of termination of a pregnancy. The types of abortion can be differentiated based on gestational timelines, that is, first and second trimester, or according to the type of medical intervention, such as medical or surgical abortion. The decision on which method to use will depend on the gestation, medical history as well as factors and needs such as travel and occupation. It is the responsibility and (should be) the aim of the healthcare practitioner to provide all the information to enable the person to make an informed decision.

You do not need to give a reason for your request for an abortion. However, a medical assessment by a medical health professional remains the advice based on a clinical assessment and history taking. Further tests may include urine or blood tests if indicated. A sonar is not necessary but may be offered if available. According to the law, the timelines for termination and the indications or reasons required to provide an abortion are as follows:

Up to 12 weeks:

- Upon request; no reason is required

Between 13 to 20 weeks:

- If the pregnancy is a result of incest or rape
- If there is a risk of congenital abnormalities to the foetus
- If there is risk of injury to the physical or mental health of the pregnant woman
- If the pregnancy will significantly affect the social and economic circumstances of the pregnant woman

20+ *weeks*:

- If there would be severe congenital malformation to the foetus
- If the pregnancy would endanger the life of the pregnant woman
- If the pregnancy posed a risk of injury to the foetus

These are the legal provisions and if there is doubt, or other reasons are apparent, a senior doctor or consultant must be consulted for advice.

An abortion can only be performed with the informed consent of the woman and no other person's consent is required. Even when a minor is pregnant, she must be advised to discuss it with her parents, guardian or family, but their consent is not required and this cannot be used to obstruct access.

A pregnant woman has the right to receive information, a clinical examination and a referral by other health professionals regardless of gestation. However, if the gestation is over 12 weeks then a doctor is permitted to perform the abortion once a consultation has been provided. The ability to give informed consent entails providing information regarding the type of procedure that is advised based on an examination, what can be expected from the chosen method, the expected outcome of the procedure, information on and a plan on how to manage pain, discomfort and/or bleeding. The level of discomfort and pain differs greatly from person to person and it is during the consultation that options for pain management during and after the abortion should be discussed.

Medical history and other relevant history is vital in order to provide personalised advice regarding, for example, possible allergies to medication being used and options for contraception if required. Medical protocols need to be developed using the evidence base and be implemented in a way that affirms the right of women to autonomy and bodily integrity and without delays or obstruction. All medical procedures require an ethical standard to be met, evidence-based information, non-stigmatising, non-victimising and non-coercive counselling must ensure that the person requesting an abortion is able to make informed decisions. The counselling should include a discussion about contraceptive needs, but a lack of decision in this regard should not result in an abortion being denied.

The options for pain medication during the procedure vary from oral, intramuscular, intravenous and local anaesthetic on the cervix. Some healthcare providers refer to what is commonly known as 'conscious sedation', where the patient remains awake during the procedure, but by using various combinations of medicines, you can be sedated and the pain blocked. Not all facilities are equipped to offer this service though. Depending on all relevant history, any current or failed attempts to terminate the pregnancy and medical history, antibiotics can also be used.

The methods of inducing an abortion involve two types of tablets and if only tablets are used it is referred to as a medical abortion. If a manual vacuum aspiration is also used, this follows the ingestion of the initial tablets, and is referred to as a surgical abortion.

There will be some bleeding and cramping after an abortion and before you are discharged, you must get information on where to go for your check-up, and what possible complications may arise and where to seek care if the clinic or hospital you are at is not open 24 hours a day.

If you choose to, you can start contraception immediately after the procedure but it is important to remember that you could return to a predictable menstrual cycle within four to eight weeks and can therefore fall pregnant again that soon after an abortion, so it is important to take extra precautionary contraceptive measures.

There is a scourge of illegal advertisements for abortions that continue unabated and many women are not aware that it is illegal to advertise medical procedures in this manner. Most of those advertising are selling pills or performing procedures outside of a health facility and do not meet the requirements as per the CTOP Act mentioned earlier, and therefore are illegal and presumed unsafe.

Some tips on how to spot illegal abortion pill sellers:

- They will not provide a landline number on any of their adverts and if they do, the dialling code will not correspond with their location as advertised.

- They will not advertise their physical address.

- They will chat via social media or on WhatsApp.

- They will not tell you about the methods they use and often offer a mixture of tablets. Some of the tablets may not be recognisable and will not have proper packaging.

- They will want you to pay cash upfront and will not have other payment methods, such as credit card facilities, available.

- They will want to post tablets to you without conducting an examination or taking a medical history.

- They will offer you various methods to terminate and tell you there is no time limit as to when you can have the abortion.

The current problem in our healthcare system is that not all facilities run by the Department of Health are able to offer the services of abortion as required. It is important to know where your local facility is, whether it is operational and what service it offers to allow you to access safe abortion timeously. Based on obstetric best practice, abortion is a safe procedure and should be available at all health facilities in the country. The protocols that guide health professionals should be available from hospital level down to local clinic facility.

There is no right or wrong way to react after having an abortion. For those women who choose to terminate based on genetic abnormalities or health-related concerns, the woman may feel a sense of loss and may require genetic counselling, depending on the abnormalities. Those who choose to terminate pregnancies experience varied emotions but the most common and overwhelming emotion felt immediately after an induced abortion is relief. There are social, economic, mental, relationship and violent circumstances that may exist simultaneously to make the pregnancy unsupportable and these circumstances can also impact on how the termination is viewed.

Depending on the individual needs and circumstance, some people may require emotional support and linkage to other social or medical services.

In order to attain the highest point of sexual health and pleasure one needs the ability to know and understand bodily functions, respect consent for sexual contact, know your own comfort levels with various ways of sexual play, know how to practice safer sex using barrier tools available and recognise any unexpected or abnormal changes and seek advice from your healthcare provider. The next section will provide information regarding relevant anatomy, physiology and disease processes which have an impact on sexual health and pleasure.

Medical Conditions

Sexual dysfunction

It doesn't matter where I am or who the audience is that I'm engaging with, the most-asked questions about sex are related to sexual pleasure. The men are usually more predictable and their concerns are often limited to: is my penis long enough? How can I last longer? How can I ensure that I can perform more than one 'round'? Most often they don't ask much about sexual health in general. Women, on the other hand, are full of self-judgement and preoccupied with having a body or vagina that is appealing and approved by their male or female partner. Vaginal modification is a massive industry and this means the market is saturated with pills and concoctions that promise better performance and the erroneously named 'feminine products' vary in what 'magic' properties they claim to contain. There are products available that are sold with the promise of a vagina that smells like roses, makes the vagina tighter, wetter, drier. The list goes on. The vagina, in particular, has been commodified and normal physiology has been pathologised with the aim to make women less confident and more likely to source products for improvements. The idea that the vulva and vagina, in their normal state, are needing improvement or that in order to function optimally, external consumables must be sought. The vague, and often misleading, tag lines about vaginal flora, accompanied by the exaggerated issue of overgrowth control, is done to make women feel that they need to buy so-called feminine products in order to optimise their vaginal health.

Women's sexual pleasure is not well researched and the bio-medical solutions are not well developed. Some of the symptoms of sexual dysfunction in women can include, to varying degrees and combinations, medical conditions and varying physical capacities that have a unique impact on each person. Some of the symptoms of sexual dysfunction in women include:

- Inability to achieve orgasm
- Inadequate vaginal lubrication before and during sex
- Inability to relax the vaginal muscles enough to allow sex
- Lack of interest in or desire for sex
- Inability to become aroused
- Pain during genital stimulation
- Pain during penetration.

Sex is still very much viewed as something that women 'give' and men 'take' and male pleasure is normalised as the main aim and often the measure of 'good' sex. Why is a 'round' referring to the period of foreplay until orgasm, defined and counted by the presence of an erect penis and sex ends when the man ejaculates? The relationships we have as individuals with our genitals, and the socialisation and strict binaries the opposite and distinct genders of either masculine or feminine set up in our society, mean that sex is still defined largely through the heterosexual experience. Fetishisation of experiences, expressions and bodies which are beyond the narrow spectrum and outside of these binaries are often 'othered'. That is, their differences, whether assumed or confirmed, are seen as outside of what is considered 'normal' and thus mirror similar fetishisation of dark skin and are seen as 'exotic'. Or are expected to be eccentric by virtue of identifying and presenting outside of the binary. For example why is anal sex referred to as gay sex? This wrongly implies that a person's gender is determined by their sexual practices and what acts they find sexually fulfilling.

In my experience, heterosexual couples are exploring anal sex much more than ever before. Many questions I receive, be it through my weekly *Sunday Times* column, on Twitter after Dark, via 'Sex Talk with Dr T', or at healthy sex parties, are interestingly about anal play. More and more straight people are enjoying anal play with prostate orgasms offering a very different kind of climax. Some men enjoy pegging, where their partner penetrates them with a strap-on or hand-held vibrator. I have the privilege of listening and assisting many couples with sexual pleasure and referring to anal sex as gay sex is completely incorrect. By insisting on applying gender labels based on the type of pleasure people experience and enjoy, wrongly implies that a person's gender is determined by their sexual practices and what acts they find sexually fulfilling.

In this section of the book, I delve deeper into the area of sexual dysfunction and relate that to some common medical conditions. The classification of sexual dysfunction is generally divided into four categories:

1. Desire disorders; meaning there is a lack of sexual desire or interest in sex.
2. Arousal disorders which manifest as an inability to become physically aroused or excited during sexual activity and sexual stimulation.
3. Orgasm disorders lead to a delay or absence of an orgasm or 'climax'.
4. Pain disorders are related to varying degrees of pain of the genitals and penetration during sex.

Sexual dysfunction is not always experienced in these very clear and neat classifications and often the issues have built up over many months and sometimes even years. It becomes a process during sex therapy to ascertain which issue came first and which component is making the situation worse. When you add a layer of relationship tension, and/or trust or infidelity issues, it can be a lengthy process of diagnosis and the related therapy. Many people are impatient and this may explain, in part, why the market for the pills, creams and concoctions is such a large one because of the 'quick fix' promise. Sex therapy is not reserved for only when things go wrong but also for sexual health and wellness. It is worthwhile to commit to the process should you want to explore your own sexuality and enhance your sexual experiences and level of fulfilment. A medical diagnosis or physical condition does not automatically mean it will have a negative impact on your psychology, sexual function or relationship.

Painful sex

One of the classifications of sexual dysfunction are pain disorders and over the decade or so that I have been doing sex talks there are themes that come up over and over again. One of the most common of these is people experiencing pain during sex. There are so many reasons sex can be painful and for medics, pain is what we are taught to treat, so you will find a lot more literature about pain than you will about other sexual health-related issues.

The way painful sex is dealt with, medically, in my opinion, is not affirming enough to those who present with symptoms related to pain. People should be given the accurate medical term so that they know why they are experiencing pain, what it is and how they go about getting medical help and advice and get back to having good sex. There is a missing link between the medicine and the treatments for conditions and the underlying desire to still have sex. Doctors and medics focus very much around diagnosis, management and treatment. They think because people have these conditions why would they be having sex. The answer to this is that sexual pleasure is a basic feeling that most people want to experience.

The medical term for painful sex is dyspareunia ('dis-puh-rue-nia') and it can occur as a result of physical and psychological problems that lead to recurrent, and in some cases, persistent pain. Symptoms may include pain only by penetration, either by finger, tampon, sex toy or penis, as well as pain during oral sex and especially during genital stimulation. Deep pain can be felt as throbbing or burning and can also be experienced during thrusting. The pain can last immediately after and in some cases, hours after having sex. Several emotional factors, such as underlying mood and anxiety disorders, can also worsen the experience of dyspareunia. Persistent pain can also lead to a decrease in libido, a decrease in arousal and also has a direct impact on pleasure and intimacy. The discomfort experienced during sexual activity does not necessarily mean the person has a history of abuse or of previously 'bad sex', however, if those factors do exist the anxiety may worsen the negative experiences and the ability to experience pleasure.

The vaginal canal contains glands that secrete lubrication, especially during arousal when preparing for penetration. If there is a decrease in oestrogen such as during menopause, childbirth, breastfeeding, there may be a decrease in lubrication making sex uncomfortable and therefore penetration may feel worse than at other times. Antidepressants, some blood pressure medication, sedatives, antihistamines and some contraceptive pills have side effects and these can have an impact on your sexual desire and, specifically, lubrication.

Painful sex can be experienced as superficial genital pain but there is also a much deeper pain felt in the pelvis and this can be caused by physical uterine issues such as fibroids, pelvic inflammatory disease from STIs, endometriosis or scarring from pelvic surgery such as a hysterectomy, or as a result of pelvic cancer treatment. The radiation used for cervical cancer can sometimes cause scarring of the vaginal tissue.

In terms of pain experienced in the muscles of the pelvic floor, vaginismus is a condition that causes involuntary spasms of the muscles of the vaginal wall and this can also be accompanied by pain in the vulva, which can then make penetration painful or even impossible.

Intersex people, whose genitals consist of not just a penis and a vagina but different variations thereof, may have varying degrees of genital structural issues which can impact pain experienced during sexual activity. Other birth defects such as a membrane blocking the vaginal opening, called an imperforate hymen, can make penetration difficult or painful, or an incompletely formed vagina.

So often women delay in getting medical treatment because, as with menstruation, where they think they should be 'suffering' through it and don't get help because there is an incorrect assumption that one should be feeling pain, no one helps in quantifying the pain associated with sex. If you've never had sex where you felt aroused and horny, you may not know what being aroused, and wanting to have sex, actually feels like. Perhaps for you the experience of discomfort and pain is what you think sex is meant to feel like.

So many women don't make use of lubricants, mistakenly thinking that there must be something wrong with them, or they are letting themselves down if they need to use something to become aroused or to enhance their sexual experience. The issue of chronic pain is a big concern because not only do you need to learn how to use other sex-enhancing tools, such as lubricants and incorporating sex toys to help you experience less pain, the psychological impact of having painful sex over and over again means your brain is going to think 'this is not good for me, this doesn't feel good, so why must I keep wanting it?'. Your desire and libido will be hugely impacted and you will probably not even think about sex in a positive way and you certainly won't be initiating it. Human nature is such that if our brain or body doesn't like a certain experience then we will avoid it in the future. Thinking of sex in this way means getting assistance for the pain from your doctor. Sometimes by the time some women do go for an assessment, their condition may have escalated from mild pelvic inflammatory disease to a vaginismus problem that has other related psychological, as well as ongoing pressure from your partner to be sexual.

Pain is not easy to deal with, and chronic pain so common, that it doesn't make sense that we're not discussing and talking about it more and sharing ways why it's important to be assessed for pain and what the causes may be. Often these conditions are curable but understandably when something is supposed to be pleasurable but is instead painful, it can be confusing. Patience is required for yourself but also from your partner and the communication around how to be creative about sex can actually lead to more intimacy. Just because you experience certain pain or discomfort doesn't necessarily mean you can't have a fulfilling sex life. What it means is that you have to communicate and find other ways of being fulfilled.

There are various ways you can manage chronic pain as a result of, for example, endometriosis, but 'tips' around this are not something that's really discussed or that there is much information about. This can apply to pain experienced as a result of fibroids, pelvic inflammatory disease, or any pain that is caused by an organic medical condition.

Here are some practical things to do:

- Have a warm bath and use over-the-counter pain relievers *before* having sex because you know you might feel some pain.

- Don't rush the process, the longer the foreplay is to try and stimulate and encourage your own natural lubrication, the better the experience will be.

- You may reduce pain by delaying penetration until you feel really ready and fully aroused.

- Depending on the position you are in, pain during thrusting can be alleviated by placing a pillow underneath your lower abdomen, or changing the position completely. In this way, you may be able to regulate the depth of penetration.

- Communicate, talk, tell your partner what you need; you need to be able to give instructions during sex. If you want to feel sexy, then whisper it. You need to verbalise what you're comfortable with.

- If vaginal penetration is the most uncomfortable part for you, find other ways of being intimate; sensual massage, kissing, mutual masturbation, use of other sex toys like vibrators, can make the intimate experience more fulfilling and fun. There are so many possibilities in terms of incorporating sex toys and perhaps kink is an option for you.

The main thing is that sex shouldn't be painful and women shouldn't delay in getting assistance for the pain experienced during sex. Remember that if you have sex during your period or when you are ovulating, you will probably feel a bit more tender than other times in the month and the natural variations in your cycle when you might be more sensitive during sex are good markers to quantify pain. But it shouldn't turn you off sex so much that you don't want to explore. Some women feel ashamed to talk about their discomfort and subliminal messaging can be at play, so communicating with your partner is vital. There is no reason to feel ashamed.

Air trapping

Many women come to me with stories of air escaping their vaginas during intercourse and a concern as to what this is. Firstly, there is nothing wrong with you. Secondly, it's natural and can happen to anyone. Many people experience this phenomenon known as 'air trapping' inside the vaginal canal that can lead to a noise similar to a clapping sound during penetration. What happens is that in the process of arousal, during foreplay, the swelling of the labia occurs, natural lubrication increases and the uterus and areas deep in the vagina undergo what is referred to as 'tenting', leading to the narrowing of the external vagina. As the genital engorgement increases, through the various stages of excitement, this can cause air to become trapped and subsequently forced out during penetration. During sex, the penetration and thrusting movements of the penis or sex toy into the vaginal canal can cause pressure to build up internally. This air can get trapped in the back of the vagina up to a pressure point causing the air to escape around the penis or the shaft of the toy. The sound created may mimic a 'slapping' of the vaginal walls, basically, 'o ishapela matsoho'. These vaginal noises are not uncommon and can occur at the peak of arousal and enjoyment. The sound will likely be greatly lessened if the penis or sex toy is inserted slowly as this will allow for the air to leak slowly. A change in the position can also help lessen the sound.

There are other considerations for this air trapping and there are medical conditions that can cause the noise without arousal. Examples include soon after giving birth vaginally – this can increase with multiple vaginal births; vaginal vault prolapse, where there is a weakened pelvis resulting in bulge into the vagina of the bladder and uterus and other conditions where the vaginal walls are distorted and allow a larger quantity of air into the vagina than is typical. There is nothing to be embarrassed about if this happens! It is a natural function of the body and an analogy of a piston pumping air in a car is a good way to think about it and understand why it happens!

Sex and allergy to latex

There are thousands of healthcare workers who use latex rubber gloves every day so that is sort of demographic one would expect to have a latex allergy because of repeated exposure. Many of them are changing their gloves up to 10 times a day so the 'real' concern about latex allergy is related to healthcare workers not people who report a so-called allergy. A reaction to latex can include redness and chronic eczema on the hands. There are powder-free gloves available for health workers who are allergic or have a reaction to latex. The powder is for the integrity of the latex so it doesn't stick together and as a result, split and break.

Another demographic of people that could be exposed to latex are people who practice BDSM. However, as 'professionals' they would know fairly early in their 'career', or experimenting, if they were allergic to latex and would therefore not experience a sudden allergic attack. Kinkmasters, kinkstresses and sex workers are all experienced people for whom sex is an occupation and thus have to look into all options when it comes to the types of protection available, especially when allergies become apparent. People who are at higher risk of developing latex allergy also include people who have had multiple surgeries and those often exposed to natural rubber latex, including rubber industry workers.

Some of the milder symptoms that can be experienced as a result of an 'allergy' to latex can include redness, itchiness, a possible rash, vulval swelling and discomfort around the contact area. If it's more of a severe allergy, like anaphylaxis, there will be more of an overall system response where a person can experience breathing problems, a swollen tongue and wheezing in the chest. A rash can erupt all over the body.

Another possible reaction to latex allergy can include vaginal thrush which can be worsened by the friction experienced during sex. A water-based lubricant can be used during sex so as to help avoid the dryness and excessive friction. Vaginal thrush can also cause vaginal sensitivity and can explain pain or a burning feeling when passing urine. Vaginal anti-fungal treatment can be used to treat underlying thrush. There are various over-the-counter treatments that are readily available in pharmacies.

Allergy to latex (and specifically to condoms) is not all that common and is very difficult to pinpoint in terms of whether the allergy is being caused by the actual condom. But it does exist. My first encounter of people stating they were allergic to latex was when patients didn't want to use condoms and lied to each other and said the reason was because they were allergic to latex. It is almost coercive and not a true phenomenological response that one would expect from a 'true allergy'. This is most often perpetuated by the male and I think a lot of this misinformation was started around the HIV campaigns and the use of condoms.

If we assume that most people come into contact with latex, either from household goods, tools and in hospitals or doctor's rooms, this means that by the time of sexual debut and exposure to condoms later in life, the allergy to latex would have become apparent by then. The obvious questions are: why is there now an allergy when you are supposed to put a condom on? If someone has a true latex allergy, it wouldn't be specific to a condom, it would be an allergy to all latex.

If you have latex allergy you should avoid direct contact with all products and devices that contain latex. Alert your healthcare provider before any dental, medical or surgical procedures to take care and ensure non-latex equipment and gloves are used. Latex allergy can be serious but rarely fatal.

Latex allergy symptoms may include hives, itching, stuffy or runny nose. It can cause wheezing, chest tightness and difficulty breathing. Symptoms begin within minutes after exposure to latex-containing products. The most severe latex allergy can result in anaphylaxis, a serious allergic reaction involving severe breathing difficulty and/or fall in blood pressure (shock).

Allergic skin problems can occur following direct contact with allergic latex proteins in latex glove products. Symptoms may include immediate itching, redness and swelling of the skin that touched the item containing latex.

Direct physical contact with latex products is not needed to trigger an allergic reaction. Anaphylaxis and severe reactions have been caused by inhaling latex proteins in the air resulting from the powder in the latex glove. Many hospitals and clinics have decreased their use of latex powdered gloves.

Sex and back injury or spinal disease

While attending the 21st International AIDS conference in Amsterdam in 2018, my colleagues and I spent time on a private tour of the 'red-light district' where our guide took us to see and experience all the aspects of the sex industry in Amsterdam. The Netherlands has legalised sex work and so 'real' business goes on in the red-light district.

One of the rooms we visited was part of a bigger building rented by sex workers and it was accessed through a side entrance in the alleyway. It was specifically designed to fit a car and included assisted mobility aids and wide doors. It was on the ground floor of a building around the corner from the busier alleys and was one of the most innovative things I have ever seen. Our guide explained that some clients have various medical conditions; some congenital and many as a result of trauma such as car or motorbike accidents. This is a perfect example of how varied and expansive the types of clients who outsource the experience of intimacy and sex are.

In the very medicalised world that I operate in, it is very seldom that patients who survive trauma or medical conditions that leave them 'differently abled', receive information related to sex and sexual pleasure. Let alone affirming sex-positive assistance. The stigma persists and it is difficult for patients to introduce the topic of sexual desire and libido to their primary doctors for fear of judgement. What the tour in Amsterdam showed me is that it is possible to offer dignified services and to do so in a safe and non-ableist space. This affirmation and access is important and goes a long way for clients whose sexual lives, for the most part, are not given priority, even in rehabilitative therapy.

The sudden changes that accompany spinal cord injury can mean that physical and psychological trauma can make people feel overwhelmed and undesirable and it can have a massive impact on self-esteem. If a person with a limiting spinal injury or mobility restriction has decided to explore sexual play, it is advisable to explore self-play in order to understand how one's body will respond since the injury and to determine what feels comfortable. What feels different? What feels good? What do you want to improve and how do you best communicate to a partner about how to give you pleasure? Open and ongoing communication makes all the difference. The pain sustained as a result of the injury or illness may be intermittent and worsen over time and without ongoing discussions about what is manageable and expected, the sexual partner may interpret the lack of physical intimacy as an excuse that may lead to feelings of rejection and resentment.

You may still be with the same partner you were with prior to the injury so it is important to explore to what extent you are able to please your partner and learn together what works for both of you. The 'spark' or desire to have sex is often further strained because your partner often takes the role of nurse as well as lover. Attending therapy sessions as well as regular medical check-ups together may help make you feel that you are in the relationship together and the opportunity to

> *Remember:*
>
> Always consult your doctor for advice specific to you.
>
> Any position can be made more spine 'friendly' or moderate by having the partner controlling the movement use their hips and knees more than their spine. The person with the back injury or spinal disease will be most passive.

Tip 👍 Positions to bear in mind: ☺

Spooning: while lying on your side, have your partner lie on their side and scoot up behind you so you're both facing the same direction.

Missionary: while lying down, place a small pillow in the lower back to support the lumbar region. Place pillows underneath the knees to make them slightly bent and to take pressure off the back and hips.

Lying on your stomach: if your pain reduces with flexion or bending forward, lying on your stomach may be helpful.

Take a hot bath or shower before sexual activity.

Take a pain reliever before sexual activity so as to minimise any possible discomfort or pain.

discuss medical options that will be satisfying and mutually agreeable. Depending on the extent of the spinal cord injury, your mobility and sexual desires, the options may vary.

There are many considerations related to your sexual health including, but not limited to, contraceptive options, safe sex and use of condoms, future fertility/conception options, the ability to carry a pregnancy to term, sexual pleasure options such as vibratory stimulation, injections for erections, performance enhancers, continuing medical treatments, mobility and the ability to have sex in different positions.

Medical advances and technology, research and rehabilitation programmes have improved, with the aim of ensuring that people with spinal cord injuries are best able to have fulfilling sexual and reproductive health. Coming to terms with the injury is necessary, and you may require the assistance of a therapist working together with your primary doctors to assist you make the adjustment and to take the lead to a healthy transition.

Sex and contraceptives

According to the WHO, in 2018, 214 million women of reproductive age in developing countries who do not want to fall pregnant are not using a modern contraceptive method. Reproductive coercion is centred around whether a woman wants to fall pregnant or not, how many children to have, what to do when one is pregnant but does not want to be pregnant any longer, or how to space her pregnancies. When these choices are not respected, and the power

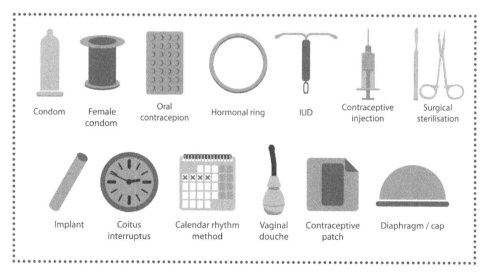

Contraceptive methods

dynamics within relationships which are rooted in patriarchy, where the decision-making power is denied and taken away from women, that is coercion. Most of the time in the development and health sectors, the issue of autonomy in relation to access to contraceptives is often seen as a health aid issue affecting those living at the global south as defined by low and middle income, namely Asia, Africa, Latin America and the Caribbean and/or rural women. Yet, in recent years, we have seen major regression in the access to medical insurance cover and to reproductive health clinics in the so-called First World countries. Third World countries continue to have the many pressures of public health systems resulting in poor access to services and ailing supportive infrastructure. When one considers the intersections and vulnerabilities as a result of class, race, geographical access, age, physical ability and access to resources such as mobile data, it is clear how a typical 'Third World' problem can suddenly affect a woman in the First World. The startling differences in maternal mortality rates in the United States of America versus a Third World country, regardless of the medical cause, the common denominator is that health systems do not reach or prioritise women of colour who are most in need, either antenatally, during labour or immediately post-partum.

The gender and racial bias of medicine is such that no matter where they are in the world, black women, people of colour, those of sexual and gender minorities or differently bodied people, remain in the margins. The commodification of healthcare, transforming basic human rights such as access to quality healthcare and dignity into services and products to be paid for by those who can afford it, means that in the Third World only a few can afford private care and have access to better quality care and services while the majority of people cannot afford to. Privatisation of services, segregation of health systems, conservative over-reaching politics that impede the upholding of human rights is more glaring, evidenced by inequitable global funding and contractual clauses including the expansion of the Global Gag Rule in the Trump era.

What is the Global Gag Rule? The Global Gag Rule, first introduced in 1984, withholds U.S. family planning funding and technical assistance from foreign NGOs, including reproductive health organisations, private hospitals and clinics that perform or promote abortions. Second, the policy forbids NGOs that receive U.S. funding from advocating for liberalisation or decriminalisation of abortion in their countries. Third, in countries where abortion is permitted, the policy prohibits health workers at NGOs that receive U.S. funding from offering abortion as an option or referring women to an abortion provider. For a country like South Africa it is important to look historically at the impact this Global Gag Rule has had.

In 2016, I authored an update of a women's health booklet for a South African NGO. Two days after his election, the grant manager gave instructions to stop all distribution of the booklet because it contained information on abortion. It has since been reprinted, and the references to the country's abortion laws deleted.

That is the chilling effect of the United States' Global Gag Rule; that 13 000 kilometres from Washington, D.C., medical professionals like me are unable to share information about my own country's laws to people who may benefit from them. The National Department of Health's website fails to list any information on abortion, the law, or a provider list. Women remain uninformed and continue to make use of unsafe means. Experts believe that 50% of abortions in South Africa occur outside of designated health facilities. Illegal abortion advertising and flyers have become recognisable on many lamp posts across the country, including at the entrance of the National Health Department.

The issue, however, is if one considers the policing of women's bodies and the entitlement that individual partners, families, communities, societies and systems have on the ability of women to be fertile and the exertion that external forces place on women, it is clear that the decision to have children or not and how to space pregnancies remains a far-fetched idea for many women.

As global and local advocacy movements reorganise, it is important to remember that the ability to choose is simply not enough for most women and that reproductive rights must be matched with direct access to equitable services. We can draw from movements led by women scholars such as Loretta J Ross a co-founder of the SisterSong Women of Color Reproductive Justice Collective and the co-creator, in 1994, of the theory of reproductive justice. With her lived experience as a woman of colour living in the United States of America and a thought leader, she sets out what 'family planning' means for people.

> **Family planning allows people to attain their desired number of children and determine the spacing of pregnancies. Reasons for this include:**
>
> - limited choice of contraceptive methods;
> - limited access to contraception, particularly among young people, poorer segments of populations, or unmarried people;
> - fear or experience of side effects;
> - cultural or religious opposition;
> - poor quality of available services;
> - users' and providers' bias;
> - gender-based barriers.

The unmet need for contraception around the world remains too high. This inequity is fuelled by a growing population as well as a shortage of family planning services. According to a study, Trends in Contraception Worldwide, done by the United Nations Department of Economic and Social Affairs, in Africa, in 2015, 24.2% of women of reproductive age have an unmet need for modern contraception. In

Asia, and Latin America and the Caribbean – regions with relatively high contraceptive prevalence – the levels of unmet need are 10.2% and 10.7%, respectively.

One of my ongoing advocacy efforts involves training healthcare providers, undergraduate and postgraduates on clinical history, talking specifically to affirming and sex-positive consultations, as well as for the equally demanding health facilities to prioritise and budget for the provision of improved modern contraceptive options. Contraception is one of the top three topics I get asked about mostly, from options available, interactions, reasons why they do not always work and fertility-related issues. The options below aim to provide insights into the options available in South Africa, most of which are privately available.

Contraceptive methods

Method	Description	How it works	Effectiveness	Comments
Combined oral contraceptive (COCs) pill	Contains oestrogen and progestogen	Prevents the release of eggs from the ovaries (ovulation)	99% with correct and consistent use	Reduces risk of endometrial and ovarian cancer
Progestogen-only pill (POPs) or the 'mini-pill'	Contains only progestogen, not oestrogen	Thickens cervical mucous to block sperm and egg from meeting and prevents ovulation	90–97% with correct use	Can be used while breastfeeding
Birth control implants	Small, flexible rods or capsules placed under the skin of the upper arm; contains progestogen only	Thickens cervical mucous to block sperm and egg from meeting and prevents ovulation	>99%	A healthcare provider must insert and remove; it can be used for 3 or more years depending on the implant; irregular vaginal bleeding is common
Progestogen-only injectables (commonly known as Depo-Provera)	Injected into the muscle, usually the buttock, by a healthcare provider; the newer ones are designed for self-injection under the skin, every 3 months	Thickens cervical mucous to block sperm and egg from meeting and prevents ovulation	>99% with correct and consistent use	Delayed return to fertility of up to 2 years after use; irregular vaginal bleeding is common

Method	Description	How it works	Effectiveness	Comments
Combined contraceptive patch and combined contraceptive vaginal ring (CVR) work in similar ways	Continuously releases progestogen and oestrogen directly through the skin from the patch or from the ring into the vagina	Prevents ovulation	99% effective with correct and consistent use	The patch may not be suitable for women who smoke, are 35 years or older or who weigh more than 90kg. You can have sex when the ring is in the vagina; the object does not impede sexual pleasure or cause discomfort
Intrauterine device (IUD): copper	A small, flexible plastic device containing copper, not hormones. It is inserted into the uterus. Newer ones are beaded not T-shaped	The copper component damages sperm and prevents it from meeting the egg	>99%	Can also be used as emergency contraception and works well in this regard
Intrauterine device (IUD): hormonal	A T-shaped plastic device inserted into the uterus that steadily releases small amounts of hormones on a daily basis	Thickens cervical mucous to block sperm and egg from meeting	>99%	Decreases amount of menstruation blood over time; reduces menstrual cramps and symptoms of endometriosis; amenorrhoea in some women
External condoms	Sheaths that fit over the penis	Forms a physical barrier to prevent sperm and egg from meeting	98% with correct and consistent use 85% as commonly used	Also protects against sexually transmitted infections, including HIV
Internal condoms	Sheaths that fit loosely inside the vagina or anus, made of nitrile, a non-latex product	Forms a physical barrier to prevent sperm and egg from meeting	90% with correct and consistent use 79% as commonly used	Also protects against sexually transmitted infections, including HIV
Male sterilisation (vasectomy/'the snip')	Permanent contraception to block or cut the vas deferens tubes that carry sperm from the testicles. It is still performed as an irreversible procedure although successful reversal has been reported	Keeps sperm out of ejaculated semen	It takes sperm 3 months before it can be cleared from the tubes. A sperm count confirms successful vasectomy, >99% after 3 months semen evaluation 97–98% with no semen evaluation	3-month delay in taking effect while stored sperm is still present; does not affect male sexual performance; voluntary and informed choice is essential

Method	Description	How it works	Effectiveness	Comments
Female sterilisation (tubal ligation)	Permanent contraception to block or cut the fallopian tubes	Eggs are blocked from meeting sperm	>99%	Voluntary and informed choice is essential
Lactational amenorrhoea method (LAM)	Temporary contraception that requires exclusive or full breastfeeding day and night of an infant less than 6 months old	Prevents ovulation	99% with correct and consistent use 98% as commonly used	A temporary family planning method based on the natural effect of breastfeeding on fertility
Emergency contraceptive pills	Pills taken to prevent pregnancy up to five days after unprotected sex	Delays ovulation	If 100 women used progestogen-only emergency contraception, one would likely fall pregnant.	Does not disrupt an already existing pregnancy

NOTE: The methods below are NOT recommended for long-term contraceptive use				
Standard days method (SDM)	Tracking fertile periods (usually days 8 to 19 of each 26 to 32-day cycle) using calendar or mobile apps and other aids	Prevents pregnancy by avoiding unprotected vaginal sex during the most fertile days of the cycle	88% with common use	Can also be used to identify fertile days by women who want to fall pregnant and can be used in conjunction with ovulation urine tests kits. Correct, consistent use requires partner cooperation
Calendar method or rhythm method	Monitoring of the pattern of the menstrual cycle over a few months, involves subtracting days from the shortest and longest cycle lengths to get most fertile days	The couple prevents pregnancy by avoiding unprotected, vaginal sex during the first and last estimated fertile days, by abstaining or using a condom	75% with common use	Caution is required as emotional or physical stress as using medication such as anxiolytics, antidepressants, non-steroidal anti-inflammatory drugs or antibiotics may affect the timing of ovulation
Withdrawal (coitus interruptus)	The withdrawal of the penis from the vagina, and ejaculation outside the vagina, keeping semen away from the external genitalia and thighs	Attempting to keep sperm out of the vagina to prevent fertilisation	73% as commonly used	One of the least effective methods because proper timing of withdrawal is often difficult to determine, leading to the risk of ejaculating while inside the vagina. Pre-ejaculation fluid may also contain sperm

Sex and endometriosis

Endometriosis is a condition in which the tissue that lines the uterus, the endometrium, is present in the lower abdomen and pelvis and in some cases has been noted to appear in other organs in the body. Endometriosis affects approximately 3% to 10% of women in their reproductive age, regarded as those years between the start of menstruation and menopause. The reproductive age is not precise and differs widely. The average is between the ages of 12 to 49. Although the hallmark of endometriosis is pain before, during or after menstruation, some women exhibit no symptoms.

Based on a scoring system, according to the spread of the endometrial tissue, its depth, and the areas of the body that are affected, endometriosis is graded into four stages:

1. Minimal: There are a few small implants, wounds or lesions that may be found on the organs or the tissue lining the pelvis or abdomen. There's little to no scar tissue.
2. Mild: There are more implants and they are found deeper in the tissue. There may be some scar tissue present.
3. Moderate: There are many deep implants. There may also be small cysts on one or both ovaries as well as thick bands of scar tissue called adhesions.
4. Severe: This is the most widespread. There may be many deep implants and thick adhesions. There are also large cysts on one or both ovaries.

The pain experienced does not always correlate to the severity of the endometriosis and other symptoms can include abnormal vaginal bleeding, infertility, bowel disturbances such as constipation, bloating, diarrhoea and bladder symptoms such as pain when urinating or blood in the urine.

It really is true what they say about the high pain threshold of women and from my years of experience so many women I see are struggling with so-called normal menstrual pain. Almost every endometriosis patient I have treated, has lived with excruciating pain for many years thinking that that is how periods are meant to be and 'feel'. Taking pain medication up to 24 hours before the pain begins, can help block the body from making the chemicals that cause inflammation. This is easier to predict if you chart your symptoms, as a pattern may emerge. Over-the-counter paracetamol, non-steroidal anti-inflammatories and prescription medication can be tailored to a combination that works best for your symptoms. Using a hot-water bottle and gentle massage can relieve lower back and pelvic tension.

There are several physiological explanations as to how and why endometriosis occurs. Research and clinical trials are ongoing and some of the topics explored include examining risk factors, improving diagnosis, new treatment modalities and patient-centred clinical research and care. One hypothesis is that during menstruation some of the menstrual blood and endometrial tissue from the uterus, 'travels' in the opposite direction through the fallopian tubes and into the pelvis and lower abdomen. This is known as retrograde menstruation. There is some immunological hypothesis that many women experience some degree of retrograde menstruation but only a few of those actually develop endometriosis. There is also a genetic component as endometriosis seems to be more common if a close relative has it.

Another possibility is that the cells in the body change and morph into the same type of cells that line the uterus and this may explain the presence of endometriosis in unusual sites far from the pelvis and uterus. Another explanation is that the cells from the endometrium move through the blood vessels or the extensive lymphatic system in the body and as a result reach different areas in the body.

The reason why the pain associated with endometriosis can be chronic is because it seemingly effects different sites in the body. It can be severe because the endometrial tissue that has abnormally placed outside of the uterus continues to respond to hormonal influences. Thus when a woman has her period the bleeding is not only from the cells and tissue inside of the uterus but it also comes from the cells and tissue outside of the uterus. The resulting irritation and inflammation caused by the blood in the abdominal cavity may also affect organs such as the bladder, rectum and bowel. This causes pain as the body mounts an immunological response to this chronic irritation and inflammation and sometimes scar tissue can develop which can also result in pain which is then not only limited to the menstrual period.

The most common reason most women seek medical advice is because the pain is often cyclical, with periods of improvement and worsening, and it can have an impact on causing painful sexual penetration. Endometriosis can affect fertility and the probability of pregnancy can be reduced due to the inflammation affecting the functioning of the ovaries, uterus and fallopian tubes. Some women may feel pressured to have children as soon as possible after diagnosis however this may be overwhelming and stressful especially when one is not ready emotionally or otherwise.

The fallopian tubes are particularly sensitive and delicate and any scarring can distort the integrity of the tubes which can affect the ability of the ovary and sperm migrating into the uterus after fertilisation. Damage to the ovaries has an impact on the number of ova produced at ovulation and therefore available for fertilisation. Endometrial tissue may also block the migration of the fertilised egg from the fallopian tubes and prevent implantation into the uterine wall.

On average, of all infertility patients, between 20% and 40% have endometriosis. The first proper diagnosis of endometriosis, for many women, is after seeking treatment for infertility after many years of failing to get pregnant or suffering repeated miscarriages. A specialist opinion and referral should be done without delay as often by the time a woman goes for a consultation and the suspicion of endometriosis is apparent, many months, if not years, have elapsed. The concern may not always be related to fertility or wanting to fall pregnant but the benefit of receiving specialist care can dramatically improve the quality of life through a multi-disciplinary approach. Based on the clinical observation and severity of the symptoms, it is possible that a specialist will treat suspected endometriosis to see if there is an improvement by using medication and not performing surgery straight away. A gynaecologist is often the primary doctor and will perform a laparoscopy to diagnose where there is suspicion of endometriosis. A laparoscopy is performed under general anaesthesia. Small incisions are made to introduce the laparoscope into the abdomen thereby avoiding a major abdominal incision. Additional incisions may be used to insert instruments to move internal organs and to inflate the abdomen with air to aid in the visualisation of the pelvic organs and structures. The procedure usually takes 30 to 45 minutes. A sample of the suspected endometrial tissue will be taken and sent for laboratory testing. The laparoscopy offers an opportunity for the doctor to check the pelvis, abdomen, ovaries, fallopian tubes, bladder and other areas of the body that can assist in grading the severity (and confirm the presence) of endometriosis.

Treatment for endometriosis includes a combination of medication, such as anti-inflammatories, hormonal therapy and surgery. Laparoscopies and major surgery consists of some of the endometrial lesions outside of the uterus being removed and this can provide some relief to the pain symptoms. Less invasive is the laser ablation procedure which removes the lining of the uterus, the endometrium. If the bleeding between menstrual periods persists, there is a heavy flow, or periods last a long time and lead to other health problems such as anaemia and if medicine doesn't help, these treatments may reduce or stop menstrual flow completely.

The fertility management options available to women depend on the severity of endometriosis. For many women the option of freezing their eggs for possible use at a later stage can be costly and is not covered by medical insurance. The delays in diagnosis can cause frustration and the many treatment options, which do not guarantee relief, can result in an overwhelming and emotionally tough situation. There are many support groups for women with endometriosis and every March many endometriosis awareness campaigns are held. It may be worthwhile to join a supportive group of friends and fellow 'endowarriors', a term often used by patients with endometriosis, to end the silence and shame associated with difficulties in fertility.

Sex and fibroids

Fibroids are also known as uterine myomas, fibromas or leiomyomas ('lie-o-my-o-muhs') and are non-cancerous growths of the uterus. During medical school, my professors used to say that fibroids are so common that some women have them and don't even know. In my 12 years of practice, besides sexual pleasure and orgasm-related questions, fibroids is the next most common subject I get asked about.

The exact cause of fibroids is still not clearly known and it is believed that fibroids develop from the smooth muscular tissue of the uterus, the myometrium, which multiplies rapidly because of the influence of oestrogen, leading to a firm, rubbery growth that is clearly different from the smooth muscle of the uterus. Fibroids range in size from that of a pea to a golf ball. They may grow and bulge into the uterine cavity, or within the uterine muscle wall and they can project outside of the cervix into the vaginal canal.

Intramural fibroids grow in the muscle wall of the uterus and are the most common. Submucosal fibroids grow from the inner wall into the empty space within the uterus and subserosal fibroids grow from the outside wall of the uterus into the pelvic cavity. The subserosal fibroids can grow large in size, probably because the pelvic cavity has more space than, for example, the inside of the uterus where the fibroid can expand.

The fibroid may increase rapidly in size or have a slow growth pattern or remain the same size. Most fibroids go through shrinkage or growth spurts. Many women are able to fall pregnant despite having fibroids and many fibroids that are present during pregnancy can shrink or disappear completely after the pregnancy. It is true that fibroids can cause infertility or miscarriages and they can be associated with an increased risk in certain pregnancy complications such as placental abruption, foetal growth restriction and preterm delivery.

Fibroids are not always symptomatic; symptoms are mainly influenced by the number, size and the location of fibroids. The most common symptoms include heavy or prolonged menstrual bleeding, abnormal bleeding between the menstrual period, pelvic pain, constipation, lower backache or pressure on the bladder if the fibroid is lower down and anterior to the uterus, and this may lead to frequent urination or difficulty in emptying the bladder. In some cases, the abnormal bleeding can lead to anaemia which may require treatment and, in fact, some people get investigated and receive a diagnosis of fibroids with a primary presentation of anaemia. There are also some known risk factors for uterine fibroids, other than it affects women in their reproductive age. Factors that have been known to impact the development of fibroids is family history, race (in that more black women tend to develop them at a younger age and they tend to be larger) obesity, as well as the onset of menstruation at a younger age.

It is estimated that between 20% and 50% of women of reproductive age have fibroids, although not all are diagnosed. Some estimates state that up to 30% to 77% of women will develop fibroids at some point during their reproductive years, although only about one-third of these fibroids are large enough to be detected by a healthcare provider during a physical examination or via ultrasound. Not enough research has been done on the exact causes of fibroids and in particular, the increased risk in black women.

Fibroids are often found during a routine pelvic examination, many of which are incidental findings meaning that there were no symptoms or complaints relating to the presence of the fibroid. It has happened before that a fibroid appears on an X-ray of the pelvis due to calcification. A complete medical history and diagnostic procedure are necessary in ruling out other causes of firm, irregular pelvic masses. An ultrasound remains the most common and reliable method of diagnosis at this stage. A specialist doctor will determine the best management plan based on the significance of the symptoms, overall health, complications from the fibroid and desire for pregnancy. It is common for doctors to delay invasive surgery and monitor the growth of the fibroid, however even if the fibroid is small, yet causes significant deterioration in the quality of life, healthcare providers may offer different treatment options. The conservative surgical procedure often used is called a myomectomy ('my-o-mek-toe-mee') where individual fibroids are removed with care to leave the uterus intact for future pregnancy. More recently, a newer, minimally invasive technique called uterine artery embolisation (UAE) is used. During embolisation, a minimally invasive procedure, the specific arteries supplying blood to the fibroids are identified, blocked off and the blood supply to the specific fibroid ceases. The embolisation blocks off the blood supply to the fibroids causing them to shrink. Multiple fibroid uterus (MFU), what a doctor will usually prescribe for a fibroid diagnosis, remains one of the top diagnoses that indicates the need for a hysterectomy; the removal of the entire uterus. Other hormonal treatments, pain management and research continues to look at causes and risk factors but there is still little scientific evidence on how to prevent fibroids.

Common gynaecological investigations to detect fibroids include:

- Trans-vaginal ultrasound with a small probe placed in the vagina.
- Magnetic resonance imaging (MRI) is often used to produce a two-dimensional view of an internal organ or structure, especially for multiple growths prior to surgery.
- Hysterosalpingography is an X-ray examination of the uterus and fallopian tubes that makes use of dye and is often performed to rule out tubal obstruction.
- Hysteroscopy is a visual examination of the canal of the cervix and the interior of the uterus using a viewing instrument (hysteroscope) inserted through the vagina.
- Endometrial biopsy is a procedure in which a sample of tissue is obtained through a tube inserted into the uterus.
- Blood tests for baseline and common complications.

I too have had my own long journey with fibroids. I was one of those girls in the school sanatorium every month (literally) to get treatment for the excruciating menstrual cramps and heavy flow I experienced during my period. This carried on for most of my teens and into my twenties. It was only when I failed to fall pregnant years later that I went for my first extensive gynaecological check-up. Prior to that, I had not experienced anything that I deemed problematic enough to consult a specialist. I always visited my general practitioner and when we both began to worry, I had some basic blood tests done and a gynaecology referral. I was still not convinced that I had any reason to worry and it was only when I chatted to my mom, and she shared her own journey with fibroids, that I decided to get an opinion from the gynaecologist based on my family history. I soon discovered that not only did I have fibroids, I was also diagnosed with PCOS. I had to make decisions swiftly regarding invasive or minimally invasive surgery to remove the fibroid and start treatment for PCOS with the aim to improve my chances of pregnancy.

As my gynaecologist explained, the chances of implantation and successfully carrying a foetus to term, considering the number and size of the fibroids growing in my uterus, was low. In the end, I had major abdominal surgery and as soon as I felt well enough, I started trying to fall pregnant again. Having sex prescribed and timed to one's ovulation cycle, can truly become mundane and feel like homework.

My husband and I scheduled date night and went the extra mile to make sex exciting by incorporating sex toys, booking staycations when possible and being kind to each other even when we weren't in the mood. We knew what we needed to do, especially around my ovulation cycle, and I managed to fall pregnant within a year of the surgery; the myomectomy was successful. I was also highly stressed at the time, working as an emergency paediatric unit doctor and was on various prescription medications and made changes to my diet as advised by my doctor. I also had acupuncture and reflexology to help me with tension and promote relaxation. I generally find it hard to meditate but during these sessions, I was able to switch off and have some 'me time'.

Sex and hypertension

To understand hypertension, a basic biological explanation of what blood pressure is and how it relates to hypertension, may be helpful. Blood pressure is the force of blood as it flows through the arterial blood vessels in the body. Arteries are the blood vessels that carry oxygenated blood from the heart to the organs and the rest of the body. Healthy arteries are flexible, strong and elastic and their inner lining is smooth so that blood flows freely.

Hypertension, commonly referred to as high blood pressure, occurs when blood moves through the arteries at a higher pressure than the normal range. If there are vessels and arteries elsewhere in the body that are clogged, or there's a reason why the heart needs to work that much harder, the blood pressure increases. This means the load on the heart increases. The heart is a muscle, so if, for example, you're running the Comrades, your muscles can only run for so long at such an intense rate. For as long as the heart is working that hard, the muscle gets thicker but it doesn't mean it gets more effective to pump the blood. The underlying cause of the high pressure in the veins and arteries needs to be identified and fixed.

If a person is diagnosed with cholesterol, then the arteries need to be cleared so that the heart and the blood can flow easier. If it's diabetes related, and something concerning the nerves and the inability of the arteries to contract in response to the blood, then the diabetes has to be better controlled so that the nerves and your blood vessels can respond properly.

Like a hosepipe (the body) and a tap (the heart), if you block the end of a hosepipe but keep opening the tap, eventually the hosepipe is going to leak. If there's obtrusions in the hosepipe, that feeds back the pressure to the heart and then the heart thinks it needs to work harder to get the blood through.

A stroke is caused when the blood vessels in the brain have a leak because they are very sensitive to pressure. The arteries in the eyes are very small and any significant change in the pressure, whether too much or too little, can lead to blindness. Issues with eyesight and reading is often the reason many people are diagnosed with hypertension and diabetes. Difficulty seeing is usually the first presentation that there is a problem and this is when an eye test is performed to test the pressure in the eye. If the pressure in the eye is high it usually means that the pressure in the rest of the body correlates in certain ways.

There are many different causes of high blood pressure and it can impact one's sexual health and pleasure in many ways. If blood pressure is too high, either suddenly or is consistently high and remains untreated for a long period of time, it puts one at a higher risk for damaged and narrowed arteries. This is the hallmark of hypertension and the damage can cause complications that can affect the eyes, brain, heart and kidneys. Blood pressure is measurable and healthcare providers usually check it when they do an examination and it can also be monitored with relative ease using machines designed for home use.

There are two types of high blood pressure: primary hypertension and secondary hypertension. Primary hypertension is also called essential hypertension and is diagnosed when there is no known cause for someone's high blood pressure. It is the most common type of hypertension and by the time it is diagnosed it has usually been developing for many years prior. It is mostly a lifestyle illness and can develop as one ages. Secondary hypertension develops as a result of another health condition such as kidney disease, sleep apnea, thyroid or adrenal gland. It can also develop as a result of certain prescription medication and over-the-counter medications such as non-steroidal anti-inflammatory drugs, Prednisone (a corticosteroid), some chemotherapeutic and immuno-suppressant meds, as well as supplements like Gingko, St. John's Wort and substances such as alcohol and cocaine.

To manually measure blood pressure, a cuff is placed around the arm and the gauge fitted to it will record the blood pressure. When the cuff is inflated with air it feels like a tight squeeze on the arm. After the cuff is inflated, the air is gradually let out. While the cuff deflates the nurse or doctor listens to the pulse with a stethoscope and watches the gauge.

The reading on the gauge uses a scale called 'millimetres of mercury' (mmHg) to measure the pressure in the blood vessels. More modern blood pressure measurement can be done with portable machines which can also be used for blood pressure monitoring at home.

The top number of the reading, called systolic blood pressure, is the force that the heart needs to pump blood through the body; that thud – the heartbeat. The bottom number, the diastolic blood pressure or resting pressure, measures the pressure in your blood vessels when your heart rests between beats. Once your heart pumps the blood through the body it needs to take a break and fill up again. If the pressure while it is resting and filling up with more blood preparing for the next big thud isn't long enough or low enough, it won't fill.

If the measurement reads 120 systolic and 80 diastolic, you would say, '120 over 80' or write it out as '120/80 mmHg'. This is the average blood pressure of most people. It is normal for some people, for example athletes, to have lower blood pressure such as 110. Levels that are in-between 120/80 and 140/90 is called pre-hypertension and levels above 140/90 is called hypertensive. It is possible to have transient hypertension and therefore one high reading warrants monitoring and investigation for a diagnosis. Although hypertension often exhibits no signs or symptoms, the impact on a person's sex life may be obvious well before the screening or diagnostic tests.

If someone is diagnosed with high blood pressure the aim of the treatment might not be to get that person to the average 120/80 because it can take years for blood pressure to change and many other factors have to be taken into consideration before merely prescribing medication. In some cases, lowering the levels with medication can mean the body is actually starved of blood and this can cause dischemia ('dis-key-me-ah'). This results in a lack of oxygen as there is nothing transporting the blood because the pressure is too low. A person's 'new' normal, if you have high blood pressure, might not be 120/80, it may be 130/90. Having regular check-ups means a doctor can monitor what your 'normal' blood pressure is by looking at vital signs and baseline readings.

For example, it is expected that young people and people who are more athletic and fit will have lower blood pressure and a lower pulse. Also, a young woman who is menstrual and might be anaemic, will not necessarily cause concern if her blood pressure is 110/70.

The link between cardiovascular diseases and sexual health has been researched and the impact is far more evident in mens' sexual performance and pleasure. This is not as prevalent amongst women and the research around this has not been extensive. Physiologically, however, there are many possible ways hypertension can affect a woman's sex life. It can result in the reduction of blood flow to the vagina and for some this leads to a decrease in sexual desire or arousal, vaginal dryness or difficulty in being orgasmic. The experience of anxiety and the negative impact this can have on relationships related to sexual dysfunction is universal to all genders.

There are various high blood pressure medications that can themselves cause sexual dysfunction but the research is again limited to penile function. Diuretics ('dy-oo-ret-ics') work on the kidneys to excrete water and salt from the body through urine. This leads to a decrease in the total fluid in the blood vessels and the pressure inside the vessels will be lower and therefore easier for the heart to pump. This decrease of blood flow impacts all organs including decreased flow to the penis making it difficult to achieve an erection. Beta blockers, especially the older generation of pills, are commonly associated with sexual dysfunction. They work by blocking certain receptors in the nervous system; these receptors are usually reactive and sensitive to the hormone adrenaline. The effects of blocking the action of adrenaline is that the heart rate decreases its beat and with less force and this reduces blood pressure. Beta blockers also help blood vessels open up to improve blood flow.

If the side effects of a medication are having a negative impact on sexual pleasure, do not stop taking medication as prescribed as it is important to discuss alternatives with your healthcare provider. Also, it is important to note that men taking prescription medication for erectile dysfunction should check with their healthcare provider if it is safe to take it in conjunction with hypertension medication.

Sexual dysfunction in women tends to become more pronounced with age due to hormonal shifts associated with menopause but also due to the development of other chronic diseases requiring medication for long-term management. Older people are more likely to be on medication for illnesses such as high blood pressure, hyperlipidaemia ('hy-per-lip-id-ee-mia') – diseases related to elevated fats in the blood regardless of the cause – and diabetes and many of the drugs prescribed for those diseases can have an impact on sexual desire, performance and satisfaction. Some herbal supplements and over-the-counter medication, in particular combination, can also contribute to sexual problems. Discuss all options with your healthcare provider and remember to make mention of all medications, supplements and vitamins that you may be taking.

Sexual desire and response varies and can be made worse by negative feelings surrounding performance, expectations of your partner and the setting in which sex occurs. Have honest discussions about the timing of sex and perhaps initiate sex when you and your partner are feeling relaxed. It is gratifying to explore together various ways to be physically intimate and other types of sexual activity to achieve sexual satisfaction in your relationship.

Sex and menopause

Menopause is a normal part of the reproductive health process and is the physiological end of the menstrual cycle. The menstrual cycle permanently stops as a result of the natural ageing of ovaries which leads to a decrease in oestrogen and progesterone. The average age for the onset of menopause is approximately 51 years of age but can happen from the mid-40s or even later 50s. The period leading up to menopause is referred to as 'peri-menopause', and the transition can take months or even years. Menopause is diagnosed after 12 consecutive months of amenorrhoea ('a-men-o-rea') meaning, no period.

Signs and symptoms of menopause as a result of lower oestrogen include:

- Irregular periods
- Hot flushes
- Vaginal dryness
- Sleep disturbances
- Mood changes
- Thinning of the hair and dry skin
- Loss of breast fullness

Irregular periods during this phase are expected and can be common and they tend to be in shorter cycles. Women can skip a month or several and then have their periods return. A cause of menopause can include removal of not only the uterus but the ovaries during a procedure called oopherectomy ('oh-off-uh-rek-tuh-me'), causing immediate menopause which can be more severe than if it happened gradually over months or years.

Chemotherapy, radiation therapy, as well as other hormonal treatments may cause symptoms such as hot flushes and can stop menstruation during the course of treatment but these symptoms are usually not permanent. About 1% of women experience what is known as 'premature menopause' as a result of the ovaries failing to produce normal levels of reproductive hormones. No cause has been found but genetic conditions such as lupus or auto-immune diseases such as Turner's syndrome (where women have only one X chromosome) or carriers of fragile X syndrome (an X chromosome abnormally susceptible to damage) seem to play a role.

In the long term, as a result of menopause and the decline in reproductive hormones women are at a higher risk of cardiovascular disease. Other risks include heart disease and strokes, osteoporosis which can lead to weak and brittle bones and increased fractures. Bone density can decline rapidly post-menopause and genital tract changes, as a result of loss of elasticity in the tissues of the vagina and urethra, lead to urinary incontinence experienced as passing urine when coughing, laughing or lifting heavy objects. Frequent, sudden and strong urges to urinate are also common. Building strong kegel ('key-gull') muscles can improve urinary incontinence but sometimes surgery may be required. Kegel exercises can be done whether you're sitting down, lying on the couch, in the car while waiting for a robot and can be performed discreetly.

What exactly is a kegel exercise?

The pelvic area is made up of bones, ligaments and organs, such as the uterus, ovaries and the fallopian tubes and they are all 'kept in place' by the muscles known as the kegels. The kegel muscles are important because of the functionality of the pelvic area, whether it's the vulva or the penis or the rectum or the bladder, as most of them are controlled by muscle reflexes. Therefore, the more you exercise the kegel muscles, the better your reflexes will be. For many women, the analogy of imagining the sensation of passing urine is the best way to properly identify where the kegel muscles are. In men, the pelvic floor can be weakened and lead to urinary or faecal incontinence. Surgery such as a prostatectomy to treat prostate cancer, diabetes and an overactive bladder, all a result of nerve problems, can also affect the pelvic floor and kegel exercises can improve pelvic floor toning.

In my experience, doctors manage most menopausal symptoms relatively well, but the sexual pleasure aspect is seldom discussed as a standard during consultations and so there is an assumption that older women are not interested in sex. Menopause can affect sexual pleasure on many levels. For some women the clitoris may not be easily aroused and less sensitive to touching, as part of the slower arousal to sexual stimulation and a lack of interest in sex may be temporary. Vaginal dryness is fairly common and is as a result of less natural lubrication and this may lead to bleeding after sex and narrowing and shortening of the vaginal canal, which can lead to pain or discomfort during sex. All of these changes can happen alone or in combination and can lead to less interest in sex.

In the majority of women, the diagnosis of menopause is made by looking at the patients' history and performing a physical exam. Some blood tests may be indicated in certain instances based on the physical examination to rule out other diseases such as, for example, thyroid disease. Routine pap smear screening should continue and once menopause has been diagnosed, taking advice from your doctor. Screening recommendations must take into consideration your medical history and risk for HPV. An 'exit' or last pap smear can be done between the ages of 65 and 70, provided the last three consecutive screening results were normal and there have been no abnormal pap results in the previous 10 years. Suggest those at low risk to have a pap smear every three years. Any uterine bleeding must be investigated. An elevated luteinising hormone (LH) follicle stimulating hormone (FSH) and low oestrogen in the blood are consistent with menopause however the hormonal levels may not always correlate with symptoms. Menopause in itself requires no medical treatment and the focus should be on improving the quality of life by managing the symptoms and other medical conditions that may impact the woman.

Treatments to manage menopause may include hormone therapy, vaginal oestrogen and supplements. To manage vaginal dryness, oestrogen can be applied directly to the vagina using a cream or by inserting a tablet or vaginal ring. This can alleviate vaginal dryness and the associated discomfort with sex. Vaginal oestrogen has less side effects, such as water retention, bloating, headaches and nausea, compared to oral oestrogen because it is absorbed directly into the vaginal tissue and does not affect other organs and bodily systems in other parts of the body. The body's own natural oestrogen can cause cancer and those who have, or have had, breast cancer, ovarian cancer, endometrial cancer, blood clots in the legs or lungs, stroke, liver disease or unexplained vaginal bleeding, should usually not take hormone therapy without consultation with a doctor. A healthcare provider must always be consulted to advise the patient on the appropriateness of oestrogen only, or in combination hormone therapy.

Strengthening the pelvic floor muscles by performing kegel exercises can also improve urinary incontinence. It is important to focus on general wellness, such as regular exercise, a well-balanced diet, getting enough sleep and finding relaxation techniques that work best for you. Many women use alternative treatments such as evening primrose oil, soy and acupuncture. More research is needed to determine the safety and effectiveness of botanical treatments. Consult your healthcare provider to ensure that you are not overlooking any possible causes of abnormal uterine bleeding from taking certain supplements or alternative products. Most herbal products are not regulated and may be contra-indicated for use with other medications you may be taking for other medical conditions.

Although women who may not have masturbated may find it intimidating to start at this stage of their life, masturbation can be self-affirming, especially as you may be discovering new pleasurable solutions you can enjoy. There is an undeniable confidence and assertiveness that comes with age, making the purchase of what could be your first-ever sex toy, fun or starting a new hobby to meet new people and potential lovers, exciting. The myth that menopause will wreck your sex life is not true.

Pain experienced during intercourse may be minimised by trying sexual positions that allow you to control the depth of penetration. Foreplay, such as sensual massage or oral sex, can make you feel more comfortable. Open communication with your sexual partners may alleviate anxiety and experimenting with erotic videos or books incorporating sex toys may provide positive changes to sexual routines.

Menopause is a natural cycle of life and hormonal therapy is not all good or all bad. The hallmark of menopause for many are the emotional and cognitive changes. It is also possible to have other medical reasons for the symptoms and one should not give up getting medical assistance nor dismiss your symptoms as 'just the way menopause is'.

Sex and polycystic ovarian syndrome (PCOS)

Polycystic ovarian syndrome (PCOS) is a complex hormonal disorder manifesting as tiny cysts inside the ovaries. Some women may develop a few cysts while others may have several large cysts. The exact cause is not known, although several factors may play a role. PCOS can have reproductive and metabolic effects; research suggests certain genes may be linked to it and low-grade inflammation has been found to stimulate polycystic ovaries to produce excess androgens. The major androgenic hormone is testosterone which, in a woman's body, is converted into oestrogen. Having PCOS means that the ovaries aren't getting the right hormonal signals from the pituitary gland in the brain. The imbalance manifests itself and can affect hormone levels such as insulin, pro-gesterone and an imbalance in androgens. Insulin is produced in the cells in the pancreas and manages the blood sugar levels; PCOS makes the body resistant to the normal actions of insulin. Excess insulin can increase the androgen production, leading to difficulty in ovulation and as a result of this, abnormally high levels of androgens can result in classic symptoms such as acne and hirsutism ('her-soo-tiz-uhm'), a fancy word for hair loss. Progesterone is produced by the ovaries, and if there is no ovulation the lack of this hormone, progesterone, may cause periods that are hard to predict and in some cases periods may be missed for a prolonged period of time.

PCOS is a common gynaecological problem and affects teen girls and young women. Globally, almost 1 out of 10 women have PCOS. I am that 1 in 10. I had no idea for many years that I had PCOS, until I wanted to fall pregnant. In fact, my only symptoms were weight gain, difficulty losing weight and headaches. All of which do not have any significance on their own and can mean many different things. And because I was never a skinny teenager, it was easy to just say, 'I have always been this way'. I have never had irregular periods, in fact my period was almost regular to the day every month. I always had clear skin and I didn't think of myself as someone who would end up with a possible PCOS diagnosis. The only time I considered that I might in fact have an undiagnosed gynaecological condition was not falling pregnant despite having unprotected sex during my ovulation period. Even doctors need to know when to see their doctor! Chat to your doctor even if you only have a few, or very mild, symptoms. You may save yourself time and marathon binge sex for a whole year! An annual gynaecological examination, even when one feels well, is important as many of these reproductive health conditions share symptoms. They can also be mild, or not cause major disturbances, but they can have significant impact on a woman's health.

PCOS can begin as early as the teen years and can be mild or severe. The hormonal imbalance can cause various symptoms and these can affect different systems in the body. Various symptoms include:

- irregular menstrual cycle
- overgrowth of hair on the face or other parts of the body
- higher levels of insulin cause patches of darkened skin on the back of the neck, under the arms
- difficulty losing weight

PCOS does not affect the health of the uterus and may affect only one side of the ovaries. The hormonal imbalance can be such that many women with PCOS do not ovulate and therefore have difficulty getting pregnant, but some women have no trouble at all. A blood test is usually needed to check hormone levels, blood sugar, and lipids (including cholesterol). Many doctors have access to an ultrasound and can confirm the presence of larger ovaries and the presence of cysts specific to PCOS. There are various options available such as medication to lower insulin levels or to help with ovulation. Even if a woman isn't sexually active, contraceptive pills may be helpful because they contain the hormones that your body needs to treat PCOS.

The most important treatment for PCOS is working towards a healthy lifestyle that includes a low calorie diet and moderate exercise as even the slightest reduction in weight can improve the symptoms and effectivity of the medication. There are various combinations of medication and some are used to regulate the menstrual cycle, such as the contraceptive pill, the skin patch and the vaginal ring. This may seem odd if someone is trying to fall pregnant, but it helps to regulate oestrogen, correct abnormal bleeding and can improve acne. To help with ovulation, some medications are prescribed to be taken during a specific part of the menstrual cycle to stimulate the ovaries while others, such as oral medication for diabetes, improves insulin resistance. Surgery is not always indicated; the quality of life and fertility needs must first be taken into consideration.

Complications of PCOS:

- Infertility
- Pregnancy complications (such as gestational diabetes, pre-eclampsia, miscarriage)
- Metabolic syndrome (cardiovascular disease caused by high cholesterol levels, high blood pressure, high blood sugar)
- Type 2 diabetes
- Sleep disturbances
- Depression, anxiety

Sex and sexually transmitted infections (STIs)

Sexually transmitted infections (STIs) are generally acquired through sexual contact via the genitals, orally through the mouth, tongue and lips, or anally. The organisms that cause sexually transmitted diseases get transmitted from person to person as they are contained in blood, semen, vaginal and other bodily fluids. One of the most glaring omissions in many leaflets or health communication around sexual health, is the important fact that some infections can be transmitted via non-sexual contact.

Some people will remember a time in South Africa when the HIV epidemic, and the health system response to it, was focused on the prevention of mother-to-child transmission during pregnancy, childbirth and labour and for a long time, pregnant women carried the stigma of the HIV epidemic. Moral judgements about the sexual activities of people continue to stigmatise and alienate, and within the views and unfair narrative that young women are irresponsible regarding their sexual activity, it makes young pregnant women particularly vulnerable. It is important when discussing, not just HIV, but other STIs that we talk about non-sexual ways STIs can be transmitted. These include blood transfusions, shared needles with people who inject drugs, blood or bodily fluids, eye splash or needle-prick injury, as is the case for many healthcare workers. The only way to de-stigmatise STIs and their associated tests and treatments is through inclusion in public awareness campaigns of all the ways people are at risk. It is important to remember that the absence of symptoms does not mean the person has no infection and therefore merely looking or inspecting your partner's genitals prior to sexual contact, such as hand jobs, blowjobs, muffing, fingering and of course penetration, is no way to judge if you are at risk or not.

STIs are really common and it is important to note that there is a difference between a sexually transmitted infection and a sexually transmitted disease. The disease process is what leads to the various signs and symptoms.

Bacterial vaginosis

The discussion on bacterial vaginosis ('vagee-no-sis') precedes the discussion on STIs because it is one of the most commonly misunderstood conditions assumed to be an STI when it isn't. The vaginal canal contains naturally occurring bacteria called lactobacilli and this 'good' bacteria outnumbers the 'bad' bacteria known as anaerobes. When there is an overgrowth of the anaerobic bacteria, the natural balance of micro-organisms in the vagina is disturbed and bacterial vaginosis results.

The practice of rinsing out the vagina with soapy water, cleansing detergents or douches, as well as unprotected sex is a risk factor for bacterial vaginosis. It is common in women who have sex with women.

Women in their reproductive years are most likely to get bacterial vaginosis but it can affect women of any age.

Bacterial vaginosis signs and symptoms may include:

- Thin, grey, white or green vaginal discharge
- Foul-smelling 'fishy' vaginal odour
- Vaginal itching
- Burning during urination

It is important to note that many women with bacterial vaginosis display no signs or symptoms.

Bacterial vaginosis doesn't generally cause complications such as sepsis, chronic pelvic pain or infertility but it can, in rare cases, lead to premature deliveries and low birth-weight babies. It can make women more susceptible to sexually transmitted infections such as HIV, herpes simplex virus, chlamydia or gonorrhoea. It can also increase the risk of developing a post-surgical infection after procedures such as a hysterectomy, dilation or curettage.

To prevent bacterial vaginosis, use mild, non-deodorised soaps and unscented tampons or pads. The vagina doesn't require cleansing other than normal bathing and douching won't clear up a vaginal infection, it may, in fact, worsen it. Always consult your doctor as they can help identify signs and symptoms and provide advice on treatment options. It is especially important to seek advice and not self-treat because some of the STIs share symptoms.

Sexually transmitted infections (STIs)

STIs are caused by a variety of organisms that fall into four main categories: bacterial, fungal, parasitic and viral. According to the WHO, more than one million people are infected with STIs on a daily basis. Millions more are newly infected with one or more of the following: chlamydia, gonorrhoea, syphilis, HIV, HPV, herpes and trichomoniasis caused by a protozoan parasite called trichomonas vaginalis. Some STIs share common symptoms, including the fact that there may be no symptoms. This is incredibly important to note and something I cannot stress enough in terms of seeking medical advice.

Signs and symptoms of STIs that may appear on the genitals, anal area or orally include:

- Pain or burning when passing urine
- A discharge from the penis
- Sores, ulcers or bumps on the groin, vulva, perineum, scrotum, vaginal opening, penis
- Unusual or odd-smelling vaginal discharge
- Lower abdominal pain
- Pain during sex
- Swollen lymph glands
- A rash on the palms of the hands and soles of the feet
- Vulval itching and discomfort
- Fever

Depending on the organism, signs and symptoms may appear soon after exposure, i.e. a few days, or it may take years before any signs are noticed and in some cases, complications may have developed.

Contrary to popular belief, there is not one 'super' test that can screen for the over 25 different organisms that cause STIs. Each STI requires its own unique test and the time frame for taking an STI test varies based on the incubation period for the organism. If you have had sex without using a condom or you have any other reason to think you may have been exposed to an STI, or you have any symptoms of an STI, do not delay in consulting your healthcare provider. Screening tests are available prior to having any sexual contact with a new partner. I strongly recommend people having the conversation with their healthcare provider regarding their individual risk.

As mentioned earlier, a drug user who shares needles is at a higher risk of contracting an STI, in the same way that someone who is having sexual contact with multiple partners, such as sex workers, are. Leaving an untreated STI puts one at a higher risk for other STIs, for example,

HIV. One of the reasons pregnant women are routinely screened for STIs is because infections such as gonorrhoea, chlamydia, HIV and syphilis can be passed to the foetus during pregnancy or delivery. STIs in new-borns and infants can cause serious complications such as low birth weight, pneumonia, conjunctivitis and sepsis.

Possible complications of STIs commonly experienced by women:

- Chronic pelvic pain
- Pregnancy complications such as increased risk of pregnancy loss or miscarriage, worsening of discharge or lesions, ectopic pregnancy, pre-term labour, stillbirth
- Eye infections when the superficial lining of the eye comes into contact with genital fluid (cream facials are not risk-free ☺)
- Pelvic inflammatory disease where the infection spreads to the uterus, fallopian tubes, ovaries and pelvic cavity to cause more severe infection
- Infertility
- Cancer. This is true for HPV, depending on the strain, with most high risk being strains 16 and 18. The cervix can, over time, grow and develop cancerous cells. HIV causes some cancers, not limited to the pelvic organs, and can cause them to develop at a faster rate

There is still a stigma attached and a moral judgement that comes with an STI diagnosis. Self-judgement may also impact one's ability to be forthcoming with the necessary information to aid diagnosis and improve the relevance of the information that one receives. It is so important that the healthcare professional receive continuous professional medical education and training in order to continuously improve patient care, acquire new skills of communication especially with young people, as well as updated treatment protocols. You can expect your sexual history to be questioned and recorded by your healthcare provider during a consultation, and a physical examination and some bedside tests such as a urine dipstick for bladder infection screening, pregnancy screening and an ultrasound to be done.

Other types of tests that could be carried out include: urine samples, blood tests, vaginal swab, oral swab and anal swab. These will all be sent to a laboratory for investigation. The window period for screening tests for some common infections are:

- Chlamydia – 7 to 10 days
- Gonorrhoea – 7 days
- Hepatitis B – 6 weeks to 6 months
- Herpes virus – 2 days to 4 weeks
- Human papilloma virus – not done regularly, however a pap smear is done to screen for complications of HPV while at the same time, a genotype testing for HPV strain can be done. The pap smear schedule depends on age, risk and presence of HPV.
- HIV – 2 weeks (for the PCR test that detects HIV's genetic material); 3 months (for an ELISA test that detects the HIV antibody) Standard tests check for antigens and antibodies (both immune markers produced by the body) and can be detected by a rapid finger prick or lab test between 4 and 12 weeks. HIV's genetic material testing is commonly used to screen the donated blood supply, for example, to detect if the donor has very early infection, that is before antibodies have been developed. This test can be done as early as a few days or weeks after exposure to HIV.
- Syphilis – 10 days to 3 months

Getting tested for STIs is vital considering 1 in 2 sexually active people will contract an STI by the age of 25 and most won't even know it. Left untreated, STIs can cause significant long-term health problems; the sooner you start treatment the more effective it can be. In the case of HIV, treatment can be lifelong. With increasing concerns globally of antibiotic resistance, it is important to stress that one needs to complete the medication prescribed and ensure that sexual partners are treated to avoid reinfection.

The following section covers the most common STIs and the ones I am asked about the most.

Genital warts

Genital warts appear on the skin around the genitals and anal area. They are caused by certain strains of the human papilloma virus (HPV) infecting the squamous epithelial tissue in the body. HPV cannot be cured and the strains are divided into 'high-risk' such as 16 and 18 strains and 'low-risk' HPV strains such as HPV 6 and 11. These strains of HPV can cause skin-coloured warts or whitish growths that show up on the vulva, vagina, cervix, rectum, anus, penis or scrotum. The warts may be itchy and most of the time they are not painful. Some people may not develop the warts, however are still infective with HPV. The number of warts or growths differs from area to area and there may only be one or a whole area of them. They can vary in size and have been said to resemble a cauliflower in their appearance.

If you have been diagnosed with genital warts, it's not necessarily true that you contracted the infection recently as it can take weeks, months or even years after the initial transmission and sexual contact to develop warts. It is possible that you or your partner may have contracted the infection years before.

Your body's immune system may fight off the virus that causes genital warts, and they may go away without any further treatment required but, if not, they can be uncomfortable, persistent and may even increase in size and number.

Using barrier protection such as condoms and dental dams will reduce the risk of skin-to-skin contact and therefore the transmission of HPV.

There are many ways to treat genital warts and these depend on where the warts are situated and how much skin they cover. The options available for treatment carry with them different side effects and costs and can range from simple creams to invasive surgery.

Bear in mind that not all bumps found on the genitals are warts and that a proper examination, and often blood tests, may be required to confirm the presence of genital warts. A dermatologist may also perform a skin biopsy.

The herpes simplex virus

The herpes simplex virus type 1 (HSV-1) commonly causes fever blisters on the mouth or face and is called oral herpes, while HSV-2 typically affects the genital area and is called genital herpes. Both are transmitted through direct contact, including kissing, sexual contact (vaginal, oral, or anal sex), or skin-to-skin contact or residual fluids on sex toys.

Genital herpes is a common and highly contagious sexually transmitted infection and can be transmitted with or without the presence of sores or other symptoms.

Once infected with the herpes simplex virus, people remain infected for life. Often HSV-1 and HSV-2 are inactive, or 'silent', and cause no symptoms, but some infected people can experience 'outbreaks' of blisters and ulcers.

The first outbreak or appearance of symptoms usually occurs within two weeks after the virus is transmitted, and the lesions or sores heal within two to four weeks thereafter. It is possible to have a second outbreak of lesions, in addition to flu-like symptoms, including fever and swollen lymph nodes. Some people can be infected but may never have any lesions.

Genital herpes can cause recurrent painful genital ulcers in many people and infection can be severe in people with suppressed immune systems.

The diagnosis of genital herpes can be done by visual inspection by a healthcare provider or by taking a sample from the sore(s) and sending it for lab testing it to see if the herpes virus is present.

It is important to use condoms consistently and correctly every time one has sex as condoms provide the best protection from transmission. However, the male condom covers less of the pubic area while female condoms protect the pubis as well as the skin around the vulva and thus offer better protection. It is best to abstain from sex when symptoms are present, and to use condoms between outbreaks, every time you have sex.

Herpes cannot be cured; it remains dormant in the body and flare-ups can be common. Antiviral medication can shorten an outbreak, lessen the severity and minimise further outbreaks for the period of time the medication is taken.

Chlamydia

Chlamydia is a common sexually transmitted disease caused by bacteria called chlamydia ('kluh-mid-ee-uh') trachomatis ('truh-koh-muh-tis'). It is spread vaginally, anally, or orally and can infect both men and women. Most people who have chlamydia show no symptoms however it can still cause damage to the reproductive system. Symptoms may appear after several weeks following infection and may include:

- Abnormal vaginal discharge that may have an odour
- Bleeding between periods, painful periods
- Abdominal pain
- Pain during intercourse
- Itching or burning in or around the vagina
- Inflamed glands in the groin
- Pain or burning when urinating

Some of the symptoms men may experience include:
- Small amounts of clear or cloudy discharge from the tip of the penis
- Painful urination
- Burning and itching around the opening of the penis
- Pain and swelling around the testicles

Repeat infection of chlamydia is common even if one has received treatment before. Multiple chlamydial infections in women increases the risk of serious reproductive health complications, including pelvic inflammatory disease and damage to the fallopian tubes leading to increased risk of ectopic pregnancy.

Gonorrhoea

Gonorrhoea is a very common STI amongst young people and is caused by the bacteria, Neisseria gonorrhoeae. It is sometimes called 'the drop' or 'the clap' because of the copious amounts of urethral discharge that drips out of the penis. Gonorrhoea is usually easily cured with anti-biotics but due to the emerging strains of drug-resistant gonorrhoea, treatment protocols have had to be recently updated, and the recommendation is that all sexual partners of the diagnosed person, should undergo testing and treatment, even if they do not show any signs or symptoms.

Gonorrhoea is spread through vaginal, anal and oral sex. The infection is carried in semen (cum), pre-cum and vaginal fluids. Gonorrhoea can infect the penis, vagina, cervix, anus, urethra and throat. An absence of symptoms does not mean there is no infection, and can appear as early as a day after exposure and take as long as 14 days to develop.

In women the symptoms of gonorrhoea are:

- Painful sexual penetration, fever, yellow-green vaginal discharge, vulval swelling, heavier menstrual bleeding, abnormal uterine bleeding in-between periods, bleeding after sex

In men the symptoms are:

- A white, yellow or green urethral discharge that can look like pus, inflammation or swelling of the foreskin, pain in the testicles or scrotum

The infection can progress and affect other organs and areas in the body and the following symptoms are also common: painful urination, bladder infection, fever, sore throat, infection, eye discharge. Anal gonorrhoea symptoms include itching and anal discharge, bleeding, or pain when passing bowel movements.

Syphilis

Syphilis is a bacterial infection that spreads from person to person via the skin or mucous membrane contact and presents with a painless sore that can be found on the genitals, rectum or mouth. The sore typically develops approximately three weeks after exposure and at the site where the infection entered the body. This is referred to as primary syphilis and a person may not have noticed the appearance of the sore because it is painless. It usually heals on its own within three to six weeks.

The syphilis bacteria can lie dormant in the body for decades before becoming active again. Secondary syphilis can occur within a few weeks of the primary episode and presents with a rash that can involve the whole body and is visible on the palms of the hands and the soles of the feet. The rash may also appear in the mouth or genital area. Some accompanying symptoms may include muscle aches, a fever, a sore throat and swollen lymph nodes, hair loss and a combination of these symptoms may disappear within a few weeks or return repeatedly.

After the primary and secondary stages follows the latent stage, where people can remain symptom free. Up to 30% of people infected with syphilis, who don't get treatment, will develop complications known as tertiary or late syphilis. In the late stages, the disease may damage your brain, nerves, eyes, heart, blood vessels, liver, bones and joints and these problems may occur many years after the original, untreated infection.

It is strongly recommended that you follow the antibiotic or antiviral regimen available and prescribed by your healthcare professional. If you're allergic to penicillin or it is unavailable, your healthcare provider will suggest another antibiotic. Avoid any sexual contact until the treatment is completed and blood tests indicate the infection has been cured. Notify your sexual partners so they can be tested and get treatment if necessary. You can get infected again, therefore condom use remains the recommended method of contraception.

HIV/AIDS

HIV is Human Immunodeficiency Virus. As of 2017, there were 7.2 million people living with HIV in South Africa, with 61% of those adults infected on antiretroviral treatment (ART). The national antiretroviral treatment programme was launched in April 2004 and due to the millions of deaths experienced in South Africa before the health system roll-out of ARV treatment, many children were born with HIV and those children are now young adults. This particular group of young people continues to be underserved by current HIV programming, which has a prevention focus and therefore leaves very little sexual health information available for those young people already living with HIV. In the instances where caregivers are not the parents of the children, i.e. many children are being raised by grandparents and extended family, disclosure of the status or what chronic medication the children have been taking is often left to the whims of people who are themselves unprepared and have no guidance as to how to disclose to children living with HIV that they have the disease and what their chronic medication is or does. Many children remain stigmatised by society in general but also by family members and this creates a further barrier that affects their ability to access services.

HIV is a virus that is carried in blood, semen, vaginal fluids, anal mucous and breast milk. The virus enters the body through the mucous membranes, for example, the inside of the vagina, rectum or the opening of the penis, or a cut, break or wound in the skin. It can also be injected directly into the bloodstream (from a needle or syringe) and from the pregnant woman to the foetus during pregnancy and during childbirth.

You CAN get HIV from:

- Having vaginal or anal sex with someone who is HIV-positive
- Sharing needles or syringes for shooting drugs, piercings, tattoos, etc.
- Getting a needlestick injury from a needle that has HIV-infected blood on it; an occupational health hazard for health workers
- Getting HIV-infected blood, semen, or vaginal fluids into open cuts or sores
- As a foetus or infant from an infected pregnant woman or through breastfeeding.

You CANNOT get HIV from:

- Hugging, shaking hands, sharing toilets, sharing dishes, or kissing someone who is HIV-positive
- Through saliva, tears or sweat
- From mosquitoes, ticks or other blood-sucking insects
- Through the air

Some groups of people are more likely to become infected with HIV than others because of many factors, including the number of sexual partners, the status of their sexual partners and the type of sex they have. There are statistically key population types that carry vulnerabilities that put them at a higher risk or predisposition to HIV exposure such as socio-economic circumstances, age, people in the sex industry, people who have anal sex, transgender women, people who inject or shoot up drugs, adolescent girls and co-morbidities that place them at a higher risk.

Within two to four weeks of HIV infection many, but not necessarily all people, will develop flu-like symptoms, which can include a fever, swollen glands, a sore throat, a rash, muscle and joint aches and headaches. This is called 'acute retroviral syndrome' or 'primary HIV infection' and is the body's natural response to the HIV infection.

During the primary HIV infection stage, large amounts of the virus are produced in the body and this is known as the replication process. The virus uses the body's CD4 cells to replicate and in the process those cells are destroyed and depleted. CD4 cells are part of the body's defence and these white cells fight infection. Also, in the primary infection stage, when the HIV virus is replicating at a massive rate and the viral load is high, a person is at very high risk of transmitting HIV to another person. After this acute stage, the latent phase kicks in and this is a period where the virus is still replicating but the person may not produce symptoms of illness. Some people remain in this stage for many decades and while they may have no symptoms, they can still transmit HIV to others. The pace of the disease differs from person to person but without antiretroviral treatment, as the disease progresses, the viral load will rise and the CD4 count will decline, rapidly leading to acquired immunodeficiency syndrome (AIDS). Because of the reduction in the number of CD4 cells, a person is more likely to contract other infections or infection-related cancers. Once the body's ability to fight off infection and disease is hampered, opportunistic infections or cancers take advantage of a very weak immune system. Some of these infections may be a sign that a person has developed AIDS. AIDS is the last stage of HIV infection.

HIV cannot be cured, however it can be controlled and managed. The medicine used to manage HIV is called antiretroviral therapy or ART, as it has become commonly known. When taken correctly, every day, ART medicine can dramatically prolong a person's life. ART keeps many people healthy and results in a greatly decreased chance of infecting others. When the viral load is suppressed, meaning the treatment is working, the CD4 count does not necessarily go up to the levels before HIV infection but the suppression in the copies of the virus circulating in the blood is a good marker of treatment adherence. Before the introduction of ART, people with HIV could progress to AIDS in just a few years.

South Africa has made huge improvements in getting people to have themselves tested and seek treatment. The success led to an increase in life expectancy rising from 61.2 years in 2010, to 67.7 years in 2015. However, lack of access to nutritious food, co-infection with TB, living with other chronic medical conditions, living geographically far from clinics, long queues and the stigma associated with the disease continue to make it difficult for many people in the population to begin treatment or stay on treatment. 90-90-90 refers to the global goal of public health systems, which is that by the year 2020, 90% of all people living with HIV will know their HIV status, 90% of all people with diagnosed HIV infection will receive sustained antiretroviral therapy and 90% of all people receiving antiretroviral therapy will have viral suppression. Even though South Africa has a successful ART programme, current trends indicate that the global target of 90-90-90 will not be met. The barriers to care remain one of the reasons why there is a continued high number of people still not knowing their status. Public health campaigns do not lead to new testing, as was expected, and the statistics show that some people diagnosed are unable to remain on ART due to various reasons such as poor socio-economic status which also makes access to nutritious food challenging, to name just one 'side effect'.

The only way to know with complete certainty if you have HIV is to get tested; there is no other way to tell if someone has HIV. Due to the way the immune system works, it usually takes about three months for the body to mount an immune response that will result in the production of antibodies specific to HIV and this is the period commonly referred to as the 'window period'. A person may be infected in this period but they may still get a negative result. That person is still infective which means they can pass HIV onto other people. The conventional laboratory tests are still needed to confirm a positive result over and above a rapid test, commonly referred to as the 'finger prick' test done by a nurse or doctor, or via the recently available over-the-counter home self-testing kit which became available in 2017.

'Pre-exposure prophylaxis', commonly referred to as PrEP, are antiretroviral tablets available for people to take who are at high risk for HIV acquisition. PrEP is prescribed by a doctor and is taken daily to

PrEP Tips 👍

PrEP needs to be taken daily for it to work. Condoms must continue to be used properly and correctly, every time a person engages in sexual intercourse, in order to prevent STIs.

If your risk of contracting HIV becomes low, you may stop taking PrEP but it is always advisable to consult your health provider before starting or stopping treatment. PEP, or 'post-exposure prophylaxis', is a prescription of medication that is taken after an exposure to HIV. PEP is taken in order to decrease the chances of the virus infecting the body. The sooner PEP is started, the more effective it can be. It is recommended to start PEP within 72 hours, or three days, after HIV exposure.

PEP is taken one to two times daily for at least 28 days. The medicines used in PEP are antiretrovirals and they may lead to side effects. Rather consult a healthcare provider to manage the side effects rather than discontinuing the PEP.

In South Africa, PrEP is available at limited sites and with the large base of evidence for the success of PrEP, it is urgent that PrEP becomes available for everyone at high risk and vulnerabilities to acquiring HIV.

decrease the chances of becoming infected with HIV.

A combination of two antiretroviral medicines is available in South Africa and it has been approved for daily use as PrEP to help prevent an HIV-negative person from contracting HIV from a partner who is HIV-positive. Studies have shown that PrEP is highly effective for preventing HIV if it is used as prescribed. Daily PrEP use can lower the risk of contracting HIV from sex by more than 90% and from injection drug use by more than 70%. PrEP is recommended for people who are burdened with disproportionately high rates of acquiring and transmitting

HIV, and in South Africa some of the most vulnerable groups are young women, men who have sex with men (MSM), sex workers and people who inject drugs. It is important to also think of exposure due to anal sex that includes bisexual people and women with bisexual male partners because they may not be specifically targeted with information and services aimed at MSM.

People who do not regularly use condoms during sex with partners of unknown HIV status, are at substantial risk of HIV infection. Condoms are effective in preventing HIV and some STIs such as gonorrhoea, chlamydia, human papillomavirus, genital herpes and syphilis.

Sex and urinary tract infections (UTIs)

A urinary tract infection (UTI) is an infection affecting one or more parts of the urinary system, namely the kidneys, ureter (the duct through which urine passes from the kidney to the bladder), bladder and urethra. Although the most common and simple infections involve the bladder and the urethra, located in the lower urinary tract, serious illness can occur if a UTI spreads to the kidneys. This applies to everyone, even children can have UTIs, however it is uncommon for men to get a UTI and this would therefore need to be investigated.

Urinary tract infections don't always cause signs and symptoms but when they do they may include:

- An urge to urinate, even small amounts of urine result in this persistent urge
- A burning sensation when passing urine
- Passing frequent, small amounts of urine
- Urine that appears cloudy
- A sign of blood in the urine such that it appears red, bright pink or cola-coloured
- Strong-smelling urine
- Pelvic pain, in women, especially in the centre of the pelvis and around the area of the pubic bone

Some women have recurrent UTIs and some sexually transmitted diseases can share symptoms similar to a UTI such as lower abdominal pain, burning urine and frequent or painful urination. Cystitis, an infection in the bladder, is usually caused by Escherichia coli (E. coli), a type of bacteria commonly found in the gastrointestinal tract. Sexual intercourse may lead to cystitis, but you don't have to be sexually active to develop it. The short urethra, which is normal for women, means that the urethral opening and distance from the urethra to the anus, versus the distance between the urethral opening of a penis and the anus, make UTIs common in some women. Pregnancy, diabetes, kidney stones and other conditions affecting the flow of urine can predispose one to UTIs. The bacteria that is sometimes isolated during a laboratory urine test is called E.coli, a bacteria commonly found in faeces. Urethritis is an infection in the urethra and because the female urethra is close to the vagina, sexually transmitted infections such as herpes, gonorrhoea and chlamydia can cause urethritis.

Some risk factors for the development of a UTI include urinary tract abnormalities which often show up in infancy because they are congenital. These can include kidney stones and an enlarged prostate that can trap urine in the bladder and decrease emptying thereby increasing the risk of UTIs. Diabetes, and other diseases that impair or weaken the immune system, as well as catheter use by those who can't urinate on their own, have an increased risk of UTIs. Any urinary tract procedure or surgery that involves medical instruments or devices such as the placement of a urinary catheter or chronic use of an in-dwelling catheter, can increase the risk of developing a urinary tract infection.

Fortunately, UTIs are easy to diagnose and treat. Common UTI disorders caused by E.coli and staphylococcus bacteria respond well to treatment and the antibiotic course is short. Some recurrent or persisting issues may be an indication of other illnesses being present. Interstitial cystitis is an example of a urinary tract disorder that can impact social life, exercise and sleep. The inability to work or enjoy sex is what often prompts more diagnostic tests and specialised management.

Interstitial cystitis is a condition that affects sexual pleasure the most and carries other symptoms such as pressure in the bladder, pain in the vulva and vagina, lower abdominal back, pelvis or urethral pain. In men the pain can be located in the scrotum and testicles, with pain experienced during orgasm or after sex. The symptoms can vary weekly or be recurrent for months or even years. Urinary urgency and frequency are also common. The bladder pain can range from a dull ache to piercing pain. Some causes include nerve problems, douching, an auto-immune disease or another condition such as diabetes that can cause inflammation and also affect the bladder.

Common bedside tests to diagnose recurrent UTIs and interstitial cystitis can be done as well as laboratory or imaging tests such as urine culture, post-void residual urine volume will aid diagnosis. In consultation with the urologist, a cystoscopy (an instrument inserted into the urethra for examining the urinary bladder) can be ordered and when necessary, a bladder and urethra biopsy can be obtained. Treatment for interstitial cystitis is mainly about symptom control. It takes trial and error to find the right combination of treatments and it usually takes weeks or months to calm the symptoms. The first stage of treatment of interstitial cystitis is to try to avoid triggers and make lifestyle changes that may help ease symptoms. Smoking may worsen pain and contributes to bladder cancer. Common bladder irritants include carbonated beverages, caffeine in all forms (including chocolate), citrus products and food containing high concentrations of vitamin C. Surgery may be an option, as well as other prescription medication and neuro-stimulation.

👍 Here are some tips to minimise your UTI risk:

- Wash your genitals before and after sex; both you and your partner
- Drink at least five to eight glasses of water every day to flush toxins out of the bladder

- Drink 100 % cranberry juice. Its acidity helps to stop E. coli from implanting in the bladder
- Urinate before and after sex; as well as throughout the day
- Wipe the vagina from front to back to keep bacteria away from the urethra (the urine pipe in women is short therefore it is easy for bacteria to reach the bladder)
- Take showers, not baths, so you're not sitting in water that may contain bacteria
- Avoid douches, spermicides, and diaphragms, all of which may irritate the genitals and increase your risk of infection

If you have recurrent or persisting UTIs, try different sex positions, use cushions to change the angle of penetration and apply lubricants to the vulva to avoid excessive friction and dryness.

Sex and diabetes

Diabetes is a medical condition that is showing a sharp increase, both around the world and in South Africa. There is a big incline in the number of younger people being diagnosed and the latest research shows that approximately 6% of the South African population has diabetes. Diabetes is made up of two types: Type 1 which affects children and young people before the age of 30 and Type 2, which is caused by bad lifestyle choices and affects people over the age of 45. Gestational diabetes is diagnosed during pregnancy and carries with it various risks for both the mother and child. Babies are often born with a higher weight but don't usually develop diabetes. The mother can usually go back to being non-diabetic within the first year of having the baby.

Type 1 is something most sufferers are born with (though it isn't genetic) but a viral illness can also attack the pancreatic cells and cause one to develop it. It is often very difficult to work out exactly what causes that type of diabetes. Both types result in abnormally high blood sugar levels. The high blood sugar levels cause damage to nerves, organs and blood vessels throughout the body, and does not spare the neuro-vascular network supplying the genitals. The clitoris and penis can be adversely affected and the resultant nerve damage is referred to as diabetic neuropathy. This can cause numbness, pain and lack of sensation in the genital area. Sexual health problems can also extend to a lack of sexual desire or libido and there may also be an inability to achieve orgasm, difficulty in feeling stimulation or remaining aroused and, in women, decreased vaginal lubrication. In the similar patho-physiological process for men, the penis can exhibit erectile and ejaculatory dysfunction.

Causes of a low libido that can be associated with chronic illness and medication not limited to Type 2 diabetes include side effects of medications for hypertension, depression, fatigue and lethargy, stress, anxiety and relationship issues.

Top 10 *causes of sexual health problems:*

- Nerve damage
- Less blood flow to the genital area and perineum
- Hormonal changes
- Side effects of various medication
- Alcohol abuse
- Smoking
- Psychological issues such as anxiety, depression and stress
- Infections such as chlamydia which may cause prostatitis and erectile dysfunction and the psychological impact of a diagnosis, stigma and self-judgement.
- Conditions related to pregnancy or menopause where the decrease in oestrogen can lead to painful sex and long-term decreased desire for sex.

If you are experiencing sexual difficulties, consult your doctor for advice and make an appointment to have a detailed consultation which should include your past and present medical history and the details of the main complaints and concerns you have. Lifestyle questions related to whether or not you drink alcohol or smoke, and how often and how much are important as they can contribute to various concerns and are not asked to make you feel judged. Take a list of all the medications you are currently taking, preferably take photos of the boxes of the medication and the dispensary note on the boxes. The doctor will also perform a mini mental health assessment as it is just as important to screen for mental health conditions that may affect your mood, sleep pattern or any life changes or events.

A physical examination will complete the initial assessment and, when necessary, laboratory investigations will be ordered to confirm a diagnosis or assess the severity of a disease. There are no strict contraceptive options for people diagnosed with diabetes as all methods carry some disadvantages and some advantages. Keep in mind that, for example, the combination oestrogen/progesterone pill is best for those younger than 35 years old and who do not smoke. It is therefore so important to speak to your doctor about options best suited to you.

With regards to fertility, poor blood sugar control is also related to higher rates of miscarriage during the first three months of pregnancy. Additionally,, some patients who have Type 2 diabetes may be overweight and/or have polycystic ovarian syndrome, which may present a set of challenges and make fertility management necessary. Poorly controlled diabetes also makes one vulnerable to recurrent bladder infections and vaginal candidiasis ('can-dee-dee-ay-sis'). Therefore, maintaining good blood sugar levels can make all the difference in improved sexual and urogenital symptoms. The discussion around blood sugar control, the options available to you and those that fit your lifestyle and are best for you to reach your overall goal, should be ongoing. Ask for more information about the impact the diagnosis and required medication may have on your sexual health, especially if you already have concerns. The doctor needs to know this information so as to assess whether they need to refer you to another specialist or a sex therapist. A sex therapist will discuss techniques to manage the decrease in your response to sexual stimulation and will include or suggest ideas to improve genital contact. Kegel exercises can help strengthen the pelvic muscles and this may improve sexual response. Prescription or over-the-counter vaginal lubricants may be useful for those experiencing vaginal dryness.

For some women diagnosed with diabetes, the nerve endings are damaged and because the clit is the biggest innovated organ in the body, there is going to be nerve damage in this area so there is an overall decreased reaction to stimulation. Also, because of the predisposition to vaginal thrush – candida – when you have diabetes, a lot of women experience pain during sex because thrush often isn't 'seen'. It can be present deeper in the vaginal canal so intercourse is painful and lubrication isn't as it should be and often a burning sensation is experienced.

Many women present with recurrent UTIs in the bladder, so that bladder discomfort, pain and spasming can make sex uncomfortable. Different positions, for example doggy style, can make the bladder discomfort even worse.

In addition, you may need the assistance of a couples therapist or counsellor if there is impact on your emotions and intimate relationships.

Type 1 diabetes is not genetic in any way, a person is born with it. It isn't in someone's DNA but for someone whose dad has diabetes they are at more of a risk of developing diabetes. It's like a family trait, like high blood pressure. That is why family history is important when visiting a doctor or healthcare professional because if there are a lot of men dying of heart attacks at the age of 50, that is a red flag. If everyone is living until they are 80, it means something different in terms of risk and predisposition to various diseases or conditions. It is vital to know the history of a family in order to gauge and give people their individual risk factors. There is nothing absolute in medicine and that is why diagnosing something has to be done in consultation with a healthcare provider; Google is not a doctor!

Diabetes and lifestyle in society today

A lot of today's lifestyle diseases, for example Type 2 diabetes, are as a result of bad eating and drinking habits. People often say they're obese because it's in their genes, but often it has nothing to do with genes; it's a result of eating the wrong food and following the same unhealthy lifestyle. If everyone in a family changes their lifestyle, the outcome will change. It's the family psyche itself with certain habits growing up that determines the future. The kids growing up in homes with bad lifestyle and food choices will have a higher than normal risk of having diabetes. Food choices and lifestyle habits start as a neonate, a toddler and in primary school and sets the foundation for adulthood. The issue of lifestyle is very much nutrition-related and if someone is eating food that they are growing, it's better than 'convenience' food that comes frozen in a container. How food is grown is important but the nutritious value of food is also important.

The issue of nutrition is political because people who can't afford good food are then, by default, being ignored and exposed to high blood pressure, iron deficiencies, vitamin deficiencies and diabetes because of the food they can afford. Capitalism has made food about class. Millions of people can't afford to spend money on organic produce and are therefore left with no choice except high-carb maize alternatives.

It's well and good to say people should plant their own food but where will they plant it? The structure of urban communities and peri-urban and urban spaces need to be looked at. Again, it centres around the issue of land. Is it okay for South Africans living in a country so 'rich' with land and soil, to be buying spinach leaves, onions and tomatoes every day in order to eat? This doesn't make sense and is unsustainable. We have to think creatively. Maybe schools can enlist the help of parents who can assist the children with extra-curricular activities. Introducing gardening at schools could be a sustainable activity that helps children on all levels especially the ones who are raising themselves. Many children don't have parents who are working and they need nutritious, good food just to be able to go to school.

Learning how to store our food correctly, re-using containers and recycling are vital and this needs to be taught from a young age. Basic knowledge of food like why not to refreeze something after it has thawed, putting leftovers in lunchboxes and learning not to waste are fundamental basics.

In addition, if parents or caregivers are bribing children for good behaviour with chocolates and sweets its setting those kids up for possible diabetes, eating disorders, etc., later on in life. Families need to have dinner together at the table as opposed to eating while watching a movie and then reaching for the popcorn bowl when the meal is done. Habits around eating are formed during childhood so kids need to be shown that mealtimes are important for so many things, not just the meal but also quality time with family.

In this world of convenient fast food, what are we all actually doing with that time 'saved'? Why not take the extra 30 minutes to prepare a meal? Talk to each other as a family, find out what is happening in your children's lives. Food centres the family and it connects us. Children are nourished, not just with food, but also emotionally when they see love expressed in all its forms.

Sex and cancer

Breast and cervical cancer are the most common cancers in South Africa. A diagnosis of cancer, the impact of treatment options as well as the side effects of medication have a direct impact on sexuality. The effect of a serious illness, such as cancer, on one's physical, emotional and mental health often leads to a change in people's sexual desire and arousal and as a result the actual physical 'act' of sex may no longer be as enjoyable as it once was. In addition, the impact on one's sexuality may linger long after treatment has been completed.

Research has shown that changes to sexual wellbeing can be one of the most problematic quality-of-life issues following the diagnosis and treatment of breast cancer. For many women and men, body shape, size, how beautiful they look and feel has an impact on their ability to be intimate and enjoy having sex. After the diagnosis of breast cancer, a lumpectomy (removal of a lump in the breast) may be performed, and while this procedure does not necessarily lead to major disfigurement many women feel an intense dislike towards their body. The gross physical change post-mastectomy (the removal of all of the breast tissue) of either one or both breasts, has a tremendous emotional and psychological impact and the acute healing process and the medicalised wound care and focus on survival may delay psychosocial support related to aesthetics. The more this impact is researched, the better the medical care that can be developed to implement future interventions that may help improve the quality of life of breast cancer patients. For many, the breasts are an erogenous zone while for others they form part of their gender identity and not having either one or both breasts can cause significant distress and body dysmorphia. Not many people are in a position to afford breast reconstruction surgery after a mastectomy and many live the rest of their lives with the physical scars on their chest with no option to improve scarring and an inability to afford breast implants.

Some women are choosing to have hyperrealistic, semi-permanent nipple tattoos done after undergoing breast reconstruction surgery. Many women don't want to endure another major surgery for nipple reconstruction and nipple tattoos are a minimally invasive, but extremely effective way to achieve the desired result. Skilled (often cosmetic) tattoo artists work with the skin and scar tissue and with the hundreds of pigments available, the areola is made to look raised in the middle and given a natural look. Surgery doesn't necessarily mean success and so the 3D tattoos far outweigh another surgery with the associated cost, healing, infection etc. Plus, because the reconstructed breast doesn't have the same sensation as before surgery, tattooing the area is usually not that painful.

Various emotional responses and intensity can impact sexual function and as such are felt by the person diagnosed with cancer as well as their families and partners. These feelings and emotions can include:

- Fear of recurrence or return of the cancer
- Feelings of powerlessness, sadness, or frustration
- Negative feelings about body changes such as scars, wound healing, hair loss, skin colour discolouration
- Stress such as chronic pain, the cost of treatment, job insecurity while on sick leave, family
- Mood disorders such as depression, anxiety and fear
- Relationship conflict or lack of communication

These are all common responses and it is not predictable as to how people will react or what intervention they will require. Some people report no change in their sexual activity and experience minimal intimacy problems while undergoing treatment for cancer. Patients may complete their treatment and only then have questions around attraction, comfort with nudity, acceptance by their partner and their partner's reaction to their 'new' body which may cause some distress. The sexual health and pleasure impact can lead to a decrease in sexual frequency and lack of sexual interest. The menopausal symptoms are brought on by some of the hormone therapies used during treatment, after surgery or radiation and those used as maintenance therapy. Also, surgery for cancers such as uterine, ovarian or cervical can result in the removal of the ovaries thereby causing menopausal symptoms. Those who are younger may experience this medical menopause as a transient phase and their periods may return.

The lack of knowledge and misconceptions about sexual activity amongst patients with any type of cancer, means that many do not consult healthcare providers. By addressing the issues related to sexual pleasure, quality of life can be greatly improved.

Sexual health challenges related to cervical cancer treatment can include vaginal dryness or irritation as a result of radiation therapy, thereby making sexual contact painful. Radiation can also cause a condition called vaginal stenosis, in which the vagina becomes narrower and shorter, which can also lead to pain during or after penetrative sex. Other treatment for cervical cancer such as immunotherapy and chemotherapy can cause changes in self-esteem and body image and may cause difficulties in becoming aroused or achieving orgasm. While chemotherapy itself does not affect sexual functioning, its associated side effects such as nausea, diarrhoea and fatigue can lower a person's interest in sex. Sexual issues amongst cancer patients are common but healthcare providers often don't address them as the focus is usually exclusively on treating the disease, with little attention paid to other areas of a patient's life. Patients and providers *need* to talk about sexual health and the impact the cancer and its treatment may have on sexual functioning. There are ways to manage sexual difficulties and issues that may result from treatment and so people should have access to an interdisciplinary team of practitioners who are able to assist on all levels.

Breast tissue also produces oestrogen and are called a 'secondary source' of oestrogen together with the liver, adrenal glands and fat cells. Hormone-receptor-positive breast cancers grow according to oestrogen supply in the body. These receptor tests are usually done as a screening for those with a family history, like what Angelina Jolie did, or in most cases, as part of medical investigations after breast cancer diagnosis has been made. It is based on this increased risk that the recurrence of breast cancer can be lessened by restricting oestrogen production in the body or minimising external oestrogen sources like creams and tablets.

Some treatment options to improve sexual fulfilment, to be undertaken with guidance from the healthcare provider, may include vaginal moisturisers that are non-hormonal which provide moisture to the vulva and vaginal opening. These are usually water-based and are absorbed into the vaginal walls and can be applied regularly to provide comfort. They are a good option for those who cannot use oestrogen-containing vaginal pills, tablets or gels. See the extra info on vaginal moisturisers in the text box.

What is a vaginal moisturiser?

This term implies there is an aesthetic product that is available to provide relief from vaginal dryness but this is completely inaccurate. (Pro tip 👍 Good old KY Jelly is not going to cut it!) Vaginal dryness and painful sex are symptoms of medical conditions, whether emotional or psychological or as a result of a physiological disease, and no so-called moisturiser is going to alleviate the underlying symptoms. The condition needs to be treated professionally. There is a reason why the dryness and discomfort is happening; even emotionally or psychologically, or a once-off thing around your menstrual cycle, but the point is that there is a reason and it's not enough to just buy 'feminine products' to alleviate the dryness.

These products are often used by women out of desperation and they go to extreme lengths to dry out their vagina because apparently their partner 'prefers to have the vagina less wet'! I've heard of women using Snuff, Epsom Salt and chalk to 'dry' themselves out. This is extremely dangerous as well as concerning as to why someone would want to have sex with someone in pain or experiencing discomfort. It is a big red flag and a moment of caution when I hear women saying their partner thinks their vagina is 'too loose' or 'too wet' or that those are signs of them 'cheating'. The discomfort is also because the use of these products is fuelled by fear and myths perpetuated about what a vagina should be like. This then becomes an issue of violence and sexual assault.

- Vaginal lubricants reduce vaginal friction in order to increase comfort and pleasure during sexual activity. These can be silicone and water-based and offer immediate, but short-lived, benefits during sex. Oil-based lubricants, such as petroleum jelly, should be avoided as they negatively affect the integrity of condoms and can lead to vulval irritation.

- Pelvic floor physical therapy or exercises promote kegel muscle relaxation (see text box below for more) and strengthening and this can also reduce possible pain experienced during sex.
- Vaginal dilators such as vibrators come in different sizes and help stretch the vagina and reduce tightness. This may increase comfort for women with vaginal stenosis who may experience pain during penetration. Vaginal dilators may also improve blood flow to the vagina making arousal and lubrication attainable and thus improving pain associated with penetration. Read more in the extra info below.
- Low-dose vaginal oestrogen cream is absorbed directly into the vaginal walls and can help restore vaginal health by improving the thinning and dryness in the long term. These can be considered with the guidance of the healthcare provider and are an effective option if non-hormonal moisturisers and lubricants are not effective.

Tips 👍

Ospemifene ('os-pem-i-feen') is contained in non-oestrogen creams that can reverse certain changes in vaginal tissue for long-term relief.

Topical emollients moisten and soften the skin. Healthcare providers will advise on the safe options.

Lubricating jelly that is water-based can also be used, the benefits are short term and may dry out during sex.

How are kegel muscles affected by cancer?

The muscles can be affected if the cancer is growing and literally impeding and growing onto other organs. This can manifest in the bladder with the feeling that you need to urinate all the time because there may be physical pressure on the bladder from the cancer growth.

The muscles can also be affected by some treatments used to treat cancer. For example, if something needs to be remove surgically, sometimes the removal of certain organs or tissue can lead to scarring, and the resultant scarring can then impede how well things contract and how well the nerves innovate.

The surgery performed to remove cervical cancer also causes damage to the tissues. High doses of radiation are passed through the body to kill the cancer cells but the radiation can also affect normal tissue. There can also sometimes be shrinkage of the vaginal canal or stenosis that follows radiation therapy. This can all have a direct impact on sexual functioning and it is therefore so important to receive counselling before deciding on treatment options.

Why buy a vibrator *after* cancer?

For many women who receive the cancer diagnosis, it is usually cancer of the breast or cervix. As these are both sexual organs it means there may be an impact on the woman's ability to feel attractive and wanting to feel sexual. Once treatment, with all its awful horrible side effects, is completed, a woman is faced with a new 'normal'. Where does she start in terms of getting to know her body again? For many women, purchasing and using a vibrator (for many women it may be the first time) is a kind of 're-learning' as to what feels good. Maybe she has a partner, maybe she doesn't, maybe she is scared that penetration will be impossible or painful. But whatever the reasoning or motivation, learning to self-play and self-pleasure is part of getting back in touch with your own body.

Radiation and surgery in the pelvic area and around the vagina and cervix can sometimes cause the vagina to become narrow or 'stenosed' and the internal 'shrinkage' can cause scars that can pull during penetration. As a result, what used to feel like 'normal' penetration can feel like deep penetration so using a vibrator is a way of finding where you are physically.

Unfortunately a lot of women lose their partners when they are diagnosed with a chronic illness such as cancer, whereas women usually stay with men despite life-changing and life-altering diagnoses. As a woman, you are more likely to be on your own post-treatment, and as a 55-year-old cancer survivor, where do you even begin?

This presents a new opportunity for women to liberate themselves because they so often cut themselves off and put themselves last, even in bed when pleasuring their husbands or partners. Now is the time to be that kinkstress! It's never too late to start and older women are usually much more confident and more able to say what they want and what they don't want. Both for themselves and in a partner. Get to know yourself and what your new normal is. Go online, explore. It's discreet, is couriered to your front door and its fun! Alternatively, there are some really good stores that women can visit, where you can chat to someone in a non-judgemental environment about the various options available that are targeted at older women. Sex toys are not cheap but there is a huge range in the spectrum and there is pretty much something for everyone's budget. Some toys are once-off experiences while others need to be purchased with the correct washing and cleaning materials as most of them are made of silicone, which needs to be stored correctly to preserve its efficacy.

Sex and cervical cancer

Cervical cancer is a type of cancer that occurs in the cells of the cervix. The cervix is the part of the uterus that connects to the vagina. Human papillomavirus (HPV) is the sexually transmitted infection that plays a role in increasing the risk and causing most cervical cancer cases. Because the virus survives for many years it contributes to the process that causes some cells on the surface of the cervix to become cancerous. Healthy cervical cells grow and multiply at a set rate however cancer cells multiply and grow uncontrollably and exponentially and this accumulation of abnormal cancer cells eventually leads to a formation of a mass or tumour.

There are more than 40 types of HPV that can infect the lower genital tract with HPV 16 and 18 – the 2 most common and high-risk viruses that are responsible for approximately 70% of all cervical cancers worldwide and in South Africa. The main types of cervical cancer are squamous cell carcinoma and adenocarcinoma. Squamous cell carcinoma is a type of cervical cancer that starts in the thin, flat cells called the squamous cells lining the outer part of the cervix which projects into the vagina. This is the more common type of cervical cancer. Adenocarcinoma starts growing in the column-shaped glandular cells that line the cervical canal.

When a pap smear is performed, liquid-based cytology (LBC) is an additional technique that is used for collecting samples in order to screen cervical cancer. The samples are collected using a brush, not the older brown wooden spatula, and then transported to the laboratory in liquid vials. The biggest advantage of this new method is that the number of inadequate slides are decreased and the sensitivity of the test, meaning true positive results, are increased. Specific HPV strains can be identified and the severity of the risk posed by a specific strain informs the management plan. With the LBC, a pap smear can be done even when there is vaginal bleeding as the processing can isolate the cells and separate them from the blood. This is extremely important to know as one should not face delays in taking a pap smear where the LBC is being used and is available.

Although we know that early stage cervical cancer generally produces no signs or symptoms, many hormonal and structural disorders of the pelvic organs and genital area present with abnormal bleeding as the hallmark. It is important to note that not all vaginal bleeding is cancer; during penetrative sex, not limited to a penis but also penetration using the fingers, the friction may cause bleeding from the healthy cervix, vaginal walls, labia or opening of the urinary tract. Sex toys can also cause irritation if not used with an appropriate lubricant. Other possible causes of vaginal bleeding after sex include: cervical polyps, infections such as pelvic inflammatory disease, inadequate vaginal lubrication, the beginning or end of a menstrual period, vaginal atrophy. Signs and symptoms of more advanced cervical cancer can include vaginal bleed-ing after intercourse, between periods or after menopause, a watery, bloody vaginal discharge that may be heavy, pelvic pain or pain during penetration. An unpleasant smell may be present and this is the cause of most of the stigma, isolation and deep shame that many women experience.

A pap smear can detect precancerous conditions of the cervix, that can be monitored or treated in order to prevent cervical cancer. Many women know about pap smears as a result of reading about them in pamphlets, magazines and campaigns but many experience a break-down in care, some at the initial stage of getting a pap smear, while others do not get their results and many experience delays in special-ist referrals from their public primary healthcare facilities. A pap test remains one of the most important screening tools for cervical cancer. Most recommendations are that sexually active women begin routine pap tests from the age of 21 and this can be repeated every year, or every three years, under the guidance of a healthcare provider.

HPV vaccines are most effective in preventing cervical cancer if administered to people who have not previously been exposed to HPV. It is a series of injections given to an individual over the course of a few weeks and as HPV is sexually transmitted, the target group on which to focus is young girls and boys who have not had sexual penetration or activity exposing them to HPV. Most guidelines recommend vaccination from the age of nine and older, with 'catch-up' vaccinations to include young women and men up to 26 years of age. An ongoing public health campaign in South Africa focuses on schoolgoing girls, however it is advisable for girls who may have read or seen information but have not been reached by this campaign at school or as part of Adolescent Young Women Programming, to consider requesting the vaccine through their local public health facility. The vaccine can also be arranged through a private doctor.

HPV vaccines are effective against precancerous changes and in 2018, a Cochrane review concluded that the vaccines cause no serious side effects. Twenty-six studies involving 73 428 women were carried out and it was concluded and confirmed from these vaccine trials, that HPV vaccines are effective in reducing deaths from cervical cancer. This was a necessary review and of specific importance because vaccines in general, but HPV specifically, are under constant attack from anti-vaccine campaigners (often called 'anti-vaxxers') who claim that vaccines can have debilitating side effects.

Once the diagnosis of cervical cancer has been confirmed, the best choice in terms of the course of action, depends on several factors such as:

- Depending on the stage of the cancer, one may require further investigation and tests such as blood tests, CT scans, etc
- Whether the cancer has spread to other parts of the body; this is referred to as metastasis
- The size of the tumour
- The desire to have children in the future

If one has precancerous cell changes in the cervix there are several surgical options for management that are available. For early stage cancer that has not spread beyond the cervix, one of the following may be recommended:

- Cryotherapy is an instrument that is used to freeze and destroy precancerous tissue. A narrow laser beam can also be used.
- Loop electrical excision is done by directing a current through a thin wire hook to remove precancerous tissue.
- A cone biopsy is done to remove all of the cancerous tissue. This is an option for cancers that are early stage and for people who want to preserve their ability to have children.
- Depending on the stage or extent of spread, a hysterectomy is often considered. The procedure will result in removal of the uterus and cervix and may be done through the vagina or through an incision in the abdomen. The ovaries may or may not be removed.

- One of the most extensive surgical procedures for cancer that has spread is the removal of the cervix, uterus, ovaries, vagina, and sometimes the bladder, urethra or rectum.
- Radiation therapy may be used when cancer has spread beyond the cervix or for treating large tumours. External or internal radiation treatments make use of a machine that directs radiation towards the cancer through the vagina or from outside the body.
- Chemotherapy uses a combination of drugs to attack the cancer cells and when combined with radiation therapy for certain types of cancer, successful outcomes are more prevalent. Chemotherapy helps the radiation work better and thus the treatments are done simultaneously.

Possible side effects of chemotherapy and radiotherapy may include nausea and vomiting, loss of appetite, hair loss, fatigue, diarrhoea, etc. Your primary care doctor can dispense certain medicines to help improve some of the side effects, including hormone therapy for menopause, which may be as a result of some of the treatment options. Most of the fatigue and weakness experienced during radiation and chemotherapy is temporary and will dissipate when treatment ends. You need to give your body time to recover from surgery, chemotherapy or radiotherapy.

Cervical cancer treatment will most likely affect your sex life because the diagnosis and treatment involve the pelvic organs and genital structures. Radiation therapy may cause irritation to other organs such as the bladder or rectum causing chronic pain and painful penetration that can worsen with deep penetration. Treatment for a hysterectomy, chemotherapy, and/or radiation therapy may also impact the ability to carry a pregnancy to term. The fertility concerns can be mitigated by advances in assisted fertility techniques and technology.

Sex and hormones

Hormones as contraception, or commonly referred to as 'birth control', is the most widely known use and eclipses other indications and uses of sex hormones such as menopause-related therapy and transgender therapy. Because of this narrow framing and outlook, people make assumptions about the sexual activity of those who take hormonal therapy, the same way that health systems cater very conservatively for the indication of birth control only and as such, negatively impacts the quality, variety and minimising of other hormonal needs of different patients' profiles.

Young women who take the combined oral pills for polycystic ovarian syndrome, severe acne or endometriosis are judged as promiscuous and unable to delay sexual activity. Many public health campaigns also perpetuate the narrative that young women are the only ones responsible for ensuring unsupportable and unwanted pregnancy and places the burden of contraception on women and prioritises hormonal coverage and access related to preventing pregnancy only. The huge gap in the information available on other illnesses that can affect people in their reproductive age leads to people often wanting to hide the fact that they are on hormones for fear of moral judgement and others, in fact, do not adhere to their treatment of other gynaecological conditions because of how they think they will be perceived.

The concern is the quality of consultation available, particularly the lack of quality information to aid informed consent. The lack of various options and choices is of great concern and has stayed with me since my undergraduate training years. I will also never forget the rushed and frantic labour wards, where I regularly witnessed health workers preparing the injectable contraception, widely known as Depo-Provera, and administering it to women immediately post-delivery, without, what I would consider, informed consent and definitely in a coercive manner. I didn't quite understand or appreciate the practice of how widespread the administering of this particular injection was until I started working in community health clinics years later as a junior doctor, where many women, both post-pregnancy and post-abortion would return to their local clinic with the explanation that they were to come back after three months. The majority of these women had vague and scanty information about the contraception they had been administered, its side effects, or what changes it was having on the body to effectively prevent pregnancy. This is so widespread, that women no longer call it Depo-Provera, they just refer to it as the '3 month injection'. These patient interactions and their experiences, particularly around the issue of contraception, caused my earliest constant agitation and questioning around the ethics of care and what this widespread practice meant for bodily autonomy. To an unsuspecting eye, these were seemingly routine follow-up three-month visits. Besides the concerns I have on the extensive use of Depo-Provera as a widely available contraception option, notwithstanding the strict regulations surrounding it in some parts of the world, its rejection by women in India, because of the side effects of the drug such as weight gain, nausea and joint pain and the warnings of the effects on the body by the FDA, the historical use of it during the apartheid era and its association with increased risk of HIV acquisition, deepened both my clinical and feminist concerns. Despite all the questions and concerns surrounding Depo-Provera, it remains the contraceptive of choice for donors and philanthropists targeted at sub-Saharan Africa.

The World Health Organisation maintains that progesterone-only injectable birth control, such as Depo-Provera, can be used by women who are at a high risk of HIV infection because, according to them, the body said that their benefits outweigh 'the possible, but unproven, increased risk of HIV acquisition'. Ongoing research about the link continues and in the interim, the WHO strongly recommends women are counselled about the possible increased risk of HIV infection and how they can minimise their risk of contracting HIV. Governments and international organisations have reviewed research about Depo-Provera's possible links to HIV risk for more than 25 years. As a clinical tool and guide to assist service providers in the counselling about contraception choices, the WHO wheel, and recently launched app, are a clinical guideline on the eligibility criteria for starting use of contraception based on Medical Eligibility Criteria for Contraceptive Use. It assists healthcare providers in prescribing safe and effective contraception methods, taking into consideration the medical conditions such as hypertension, epilepsy, HIV or medically relevant characteristics such as taking Warfarin. The wheel includes recommendations on initiating use of the nine common types of contraceptive methods.

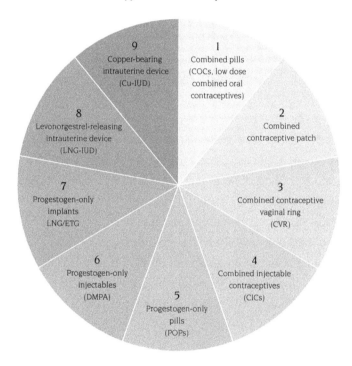

One commonality amongst women in South Africa, and women generally, is that most don't receive comprehensive sexual education and therefore don't understand our bodies properly. With a very low health literacy, women, despite being well-versed in other aspects of life and career are still at risk of myth-laden knowledge about their bodies, vaginal health, birthing processes, sexual pleasure, and therefore rely on health professionals to provide us with information. Many women are not confident enough to question their healthcare providers and the power dynamics in the consultation room foster infantalisation and, in the process, is disempowering women. Due to a lack of continued medical education and training, specific to sexual and reproductive health, health workers are not always geared or prepared for comprehensive discussions on transition therapy, side effects of contraception, the links to sexual pleasure, and other personal reasons why patients may opt for one method over another.

Many transgender women self-medicate and have no reliable health providers or clinics they can depend on for continuous care and support. Transgender women use different combinations of hormones with the aim to assist in the development of female secondary sex characteristics, with minimisation of male secondary sex characteristics. In keeping with the Tanner stages of development (named after Professor James Tanner, who was the first to identify the visible stages of puberty), various bodily changes can be expected. Breast development, usually to Tanner stage 2 or 3, redistribution of facial and body subcutaneous fat, reduction of muscle mass, reduction of body hair and facial hair and changes in sweat and odour. Sexual organ and gland effects of feminisation therapy may include a reduction in erectile function, changes in libido, reduced or absent sperm count and ejaculatory fluid, and reduced testicular size. Generally, the initial consultation will include a wellness check-up so that the baseline results assist with monitoring once hormonal treatment is started.

The type of oestrogen used for feminising therapy is a 'bioidentical' hormone in that it is chemically identical to that from a human ovary. The mode of delivery most common and available in South Africa for transgender women is a transdermal patch, oral or sublingual tablet. Suppression of testosterone production and blocking of its effects leads to the minimisation of male secondary sexual characteristics and is prescribed with care. It is important to manage the expectations of what oestrogen therapy can achieve as unfortunately many of the male characteristics are not one hundred per cent irreversible post-puberty. Laboratory monitoring for feminising hormone therapy at different intervals is recommended and under the guidance of a healthcare provider.

When preparing for your next consultation there are a few points to keep in mind. These tips will help you become an advocate for yourself in order to optimise your care.

- Compile a list of the questions you have for your health pro-vider and remember to take this with to your next appointment.
- Keep track of your cycle, such as the number of days you have a bleed, the presence of clots, any associated pain, the first day of your bleed.
- Ask questions about the different contraceptive methods avail-able to you and their 'failure rates', or how often they have been shown not to work as well and what circumstances make them not work effectively.
- Ask about the signs and symptoms of pregnancy.
- Talk to your healthcare provider about the factors that might make it hard for you to regularly use a contraceptive. This can help you decide whether your lifestyle is better suited to taking daily pills, or if you should consider an IUD that could prevent pregnancies for multiple years.
- Find out what kind of medical conditions run in your family. You may be certain of your own medical history, but you'll want to be able to tell your healthcare provider if your family has a his-tory of, for instance, cancer, blood disorders or cardiovascular events such as strokes.
- Be honest about your use of alcohol, smoking and herbal detoxifiers, usually dried and produced from parts of the plant, including seeds, bark, roots and fruits. It is important to acknowledge your use (perhaps somewhat reluctantly) of any of these to avoid risks associated with them while on particular contraceptive methods.
- If your healthcare provider does not ask specific questions about sexual pleasure, or about your medical conditions or

medication which may have an impact your ability to enjoy sex, be honest about your experience, rather than stopping your treatment.

Hormonal Preparations: Sex Hormones

Natural hormonal therapy and synthetic hormonal therapy:

- Oestrogen
- Progesterone
- Testosterone

Mode of delivery:

- Oral pill
- Patch
- Topical
- Vaginal
- Injectable
- Intra-uterine

Various roles/stages sexual and reproductive development:

- Puberty
- Pregnancy
- Menopause (peri-menopause, post-menopause)
- Sexual dysfunction
- Contraception
- Transgender health (feminising therapy and masculinising therapy)
- Gynaecological conditions (menstrual regulation, endometriosis treatment, PCOS management)

Abstinence

Sex, and what counts as sex, if you think of 'outercourse' versus 'intercourse' and sexual contact that does not involve penetration of the vagina or anus by a penis, throws the definition open to interpretation. Therefore, the definition of abstinence means different things to different people. Many people agree on the definition of abstinence as not having any kind of sexual contact with another person, including vaginal, oral, and anal sex. Masturbation is self-play and carries no risk of pregnancy or sexual disease and it follows that one can abstain from sex but enjoy self-pleasure or masturbation.

'Outercourse' is sexual contact with another person with clothes on, such as dry humping. Provided there is no contact with sperm it is more effective in preventing pregnancy than, for example, thigh sex or 'ukusoma'. Pre-cum semen can still get into the vagina from ejaculating on the thighs and some STIs can also still be transmitted. Genital rubbing, without penetration or the presence of fluids, can still transmit HPV and herpes through the skin rubbing on the genitals without the presence of a discharge even when blisters are not visible. This mostly occurs during the first 12 months of herpes infections.

The vaginal fluids and semen that can be present on hands, can through oral sex and/or anal sex, still carry a risk of STDs, so use a condom, finger cots (individual latex coverings for fingers) and dental dams during oral sex and anal sex. Oral sex won't lead to pregnancy; however it is important to remember that sperm can get into the vagina even during anal sex.

People do not always have cultural or religious pressure to abstain but it can be a healthy choice for young adults who have never had sex before. Encouraging the delay of the first penetrative sexual contact for oneself and, as we know many parents wish as much for their children, does, I believe, foster society's obsession with 'purity' and virginity pledges. A more affirming stance, especially regarding young women's sexual expression and pleasure must be adopted. Celibacy is associated with abstinence due to religious or spiritual reasons but there are so many reasons to abstain. Break-ups can cause some people to wish for more time to get over a lover or a relationship, or sadly, as part of bereavement from the death of a partner. Your healthcare provider may advise you to avoid sexual contact post-surgery, while getting treatment for infection or during recovery from illness.

I always recommend using a reliable contraceptive that does not rely on willpower because I have been in the field long enough to tell you that causal sex, one-night stands, 'monate wa letswai' and the heat, can take over and it *does* take over and therefore exposure to STIs and chance of falling pregnant are high. It is also important to assist young people in getting comfortable purchasing condoms and normalising young women carrying condoms.

Research has shown that many people do not use a barrier method, that is, the male or internal condom, properly and consistently with every sexual contact. As recent as 2016, the South Africa Demographic and Health Survey showed that in adults aged 15 to 49, 17% of men and 5% of women reported having two or more sexual partners in the previous 12 months. Inadequate condom use during the last sexual intercourse was reported among 58% of women and 65% of men, who had had multiple partners in the past year. Many teenagers were born with HIV and they are often a forgotten population group as most of the programming tends to focus on abstinence to avoid new infections and not enough on comprehensive non-judgemental sexuality information. On the wellness episode of 'Sex Talk with Dr T' on DSTV, I hosted a young man who shared his journey with HIV with full disclosure, acceptance and adherence to his treatment. He described the complexities that caregivers and parents face regarding disclosure of the child's status when they start questioning and demonstrating cognitive abilities to understand the disease process and the details of the daily treatment regimen.

It is important to remember that young people spend many hours in school and therefore teachers require the training and personal development to assist their students with the tools to provide sexual health information that is empowering to learners. The content, as well as the delivery methods, are important and should deal with emotional aspects of sexual health, contraception, negotiating condom use, STIs, unsupportable pregnancies and constitutional rights of minors related to sexual health and well-being. The crisis levels of sexual assault and rape in our country means that access to post-trauma centres for immediate emergency contraception and post-exposure prophylaxis for HIV transmission should be guaranteed.

Tip 👍 **A word on condoms from Dr T:**

The storage of condoms is important so in order to keep the integrity of the condom store them in a cool, dry place and away from sunlight.

Don't keep them anywhere they'll be exposed to heat or fluctuations in temperatures, including your cubbyhole, wallet, or back pocket.

Do not reuse the same condom for oral, vaginal or anal sex.

A condom can prevent STDs, pregnancy, and there are lubricants that can be bought to enhance pleasure.

Bereavement

Bereavement is the process of dealing with the loss of someone important. The process can take time in adjusting to the fact that the partner you had is either not there or has passed away, and that there has been a major shift in the way the relationship once was. Sex is of course one of the casualties in this loss.

Older people, especially older women in conservative African societies, still have to wear specific clothing for a certain period of time when their husband passes. There is a societal expectation that she needs to be seen to be in mourning and people must see that she is a widow, whereas those cultural practices are not in place for men. There are so many myths surrounding a woman who has lost her husband, like the belief that she has bad spirits following her, that it goes so far as men must know not to approach her because she is a recent widow. This again speaks to the pressures of our time and the context that women have to navigate around their own sexuality. The truth is that women are judged more harshly for moving on. Whether it is moving homes, taking off a ring or going on dates, women are generally more criticised.

Sexual dysfunction in older women isn't researched in the same way that sexual dysfunction in men is. Pharmaceutical developments and technology don't focus on hormone assistance or sexual pleasure tools for women. This speaks to the bias of medicine; the penis and male pleasure being more prized than women's.

A lot of conversations I have with older women is around how liberated they feel at an older age because they 'own' their own person and no longer feel that they need to act in a certain way to please their families or their partner or society. They find they are able to have sex in the ways that they want. Casual sex is not a young people thing; older people find it affirming to be able to have short-term relationships with people that are very clear in terms of what is expected from both parties.

Of course, losing a partner, whether you are young or old, is one of the hardest things people face in life and as the one who is left behind you may have a deep bond with the deceased for many years. That relationship can remain a central aspect of your life.

The stages of grief are shock and disbelief, especially in the acute time; denial; anger and guilt and over time these emotions can develop into states of depression or even mood disorders. Eventually some kind of normalcy or routine may be established without that partner, and hopefully a kind of acceptance. Until you get to that place where you are okay and you have accepted the fact that your partner has passed on, there is not much room in wanting to explore relationships with other people.

I've had clients in therapy who, although they don't want to be engaged or available emotionally for someone else as they feel they still owe that emotional connection to their partner, some of them engage in casual sex that doesn't have any deep meaning for them. It is important to recognise that people grieve differently. Whatever ideas people have around their sexuality and sexual pleasure are valid. There are no set feelings or an order of how you experience grief, and it's not a once-off event. Grief has its ebbs and flows.

There will be many difficult 'firsts' you'll experience without your partner and sometimes there are children involved. You might feel fine, until say, your child is in matric but then you might struggle with your partner not being there for that big milestone. Unfortunately friends and family can become a bit impatient as you go through this period of trying to work through the loss of someone.

Some people may never want to date again after their partner has passed; some people make certain vows that they take seriously such as to maintain fidelity to the deceased person for as long as they are alive. The guilt that comes when a partner does pass away – you are the surviving partner and want to start dating again – is another aspect of bereavement.

It can take a while to accept that they may be breaking the vow they made to the deceased and they might not be fully intimate with the new partner until they have forgiven and accepted themselves in that way.

Finding a new lover may not necessarily be something that they are interested in. I always keep an open mind; help people with the kind of sex they want to have and with who they want to have it with. There isn't any scripted sexual pleasure that people must experience; it's what people want, when they want it, and how they want it. My role is to affirm people's healthy sexual behaviour. Emotionally, people may still be vulnerable and even though you feel ready to start dating again, the issue of communication is important. As you go back into the dating game, you need to tell people that you are going through bereavement and have a specific type of vulnerability because rejection can make anxiety worse and trigger the despair of being alone again. It is possible to enter into a new and meaningful relationship without denying the feelings or minimising the importance of your previous relationship. Even if someone didn't die, there can be life-altering events that caused the relationship to end and it is okay to still celebrate what was. People don't need to feel the pressure to deny their previous experiences or minimise them in any way.

The issue of intimacy is the one that causes the most apprehension and uneasiness because often the fear of allowing another person into your life, and worrying about losing them if they also die or leave can be debilitating in terms of moving forward. It is a vicious cycle as you don't want to start relationships and you avoid going on dates because of the fear of losing someone again.

People may experience difficulties with arousal and performance when entering new relationships and because grief is so deeply personal we shouldn't over-medicalise or depend too much on pharmaceutical solutions when the underlying problems can be psychological or seasonal.

I go through a bit of a mood disturbance every December where my grief is not related to a partner or someone I had a sexual relationship with, but to my dad. He died on Christmas day, so every year I feel down around that time and the feeling lingers after Christmas and into the New Year. It was only this year, 2019, that I realised my feelings are related to my dad's death and I was then able to process it. Often one can anticipate certain mood changes but they can be very mild and you therefore don't always have the insight to process them correctly.

While there is a place for pharmaceutical solutions when it comes to grief, I think it's affirming for people to understand what the pattern is to their grief and where it comes from. That way you can cope better when you know that something's coming, get support and share with people what you're going through. When people are in new relationships they may find intimacy and sex difficult around the time of the event but it is important they don't minimise that event and the effect it has on them. Talking to your new partner can contribute to intimacy as it can bring people closer together. In my case, my feelings about losing my dad impacted my ability to have fun and be happy, so not talking about your loss can have an impact on your sex life. Relationships are key and how you talk about intimacy has to be about more than the person you are having sex with and be about building a healthy environment for communication, trust and vulnerability. There are people who have sex with multiple partners and for them intimacy might look very different. Those relationships may also look very different in what is important to them.

It *is* possible to resume sexual activity after you've been celibate for a while. Some women have certain rules to live by during the mourning period but after that period is over, they need to be asked how they are and what their fears and anxieties are for their new life. Women are often expected to not want to have sex anyway so when you are an older woman, who is also a widow, no one actually prioritises the fact that sex may be an option. I'm the biggest mascot for self-pleasure and self-play so I will always advocate that for anyone who is trying to have sex again after a difficult time. To ease back into erotic experiences, self-pleasure and self-affirmation is a really positive thing, and it will also help you learn what your body responds to as your brain might not respond to the same things as before, and certain things may remind you of the partner you are trying to get over. You can have self-play without penetration, and what is important is whatever is comfortable for you until you are ready. Foreplay is as important because if you've decided in your new relationship that you're not going to be using sex toys, there is so much you can do that will improve intimacy and make the other person feel understood and heard.

The pressure, again, to go from no sex to a full-on experimental sexual goddess, I find to be an unfair expectation. Take it one step at a time, and if you really feel like it and it is what you want to do, then go for it. Communication is key, whether it's with a new dating partner or a casual sex partner, they need to understand the experiences of your previous relationships. If they don't know what you have had to deal with, they may not pre-empt certain things and it may be frustrating when they think they are showing respect in a certain way but receive a different response from you. Communication will help in understanding why certain people have certain boundaries and why creating safer spaces will lead to being more intimate with your partner and having more fulfilling sexual experiences. Texting, sexting, phoning and emailing, can help in escalating things quite quickly. The expectations of returning calls and texts is also important. Dating apps can be used and it is important to explore and find out what excites you and allow yourself to be surprised and not tie yourself to a previous script. Many people who have lost their partners from long-term relationships may not have had the best sex life, so this is a chance to have the sex that they've always wanted to have.

In terms of families, you need to determine what aspects of your relationship you want to share. If there are children involved and you are comfortable with your new lover or partner, then decide when the appropriate time is to introduce them to your children. This is not sex-related, per se, but it does influence your sexual ability in terms of the logistics of who visits who, where to have sex, etc. Boundaries will shift and change as the relationship progresses; it will stop feeling like hard work. Unless you are committed to being open and honest from the beginning, you will never get to a stage where you feel fulfilled and develop that trust. Boundaries are important because whether you are in a casual or serious relationship, it's important to listen and respect other people in your choices. Get help, speak to a bereavement counsellor or join a support group. Often other people can't imagine what you might be going through and your sexual partner isn't necessarily the person helping you through your grief. Sometimes it is actually better for it not to be the same person as you need to grieve and perhaps cry in a safe space and then come back and be sexual with your new partner.

Bereavement in terms of women dealing with loss as a result of a miscarriage or an induced abortion carries with it huge implications. There is often an expectation around women who choose to end a pregnancy, that because they were pregnant and chose to have an abortion, that they will be turned off sex. That is not true. What is true, though, is that women have many reasons as to why they do not want to be pregnant anymore and therefore choose to terminate their pregnancy. Sometimes the reasons can be tragic but the focus so often tends to be on how women feel after the abortion, i.e. they are feeling sad only because of having the abortion. For many women the overwhelming feeling is relief.

Not enough time is spent with women who feel that they can't have a child. People often only concentrate on the feeling of loss and sadness after an abortion but there are reasons and situations that made that woman feel that she couldn't support a pregnancy in the first place. There's a lot of research done but a lot of it doesn't support the existence of post-abortion depression and much of mainstream media, blogs and support groups try to push this idea. This often comes across as anti-choice and is used as a weapon to convince women not to have an abortion by citing depression and trauma as a lifelong consequence. This is incredibly unfair, especially in a country like South Africa where the trauma surrounding abortion stems from women not having access to adequate and safe healthcare facilities. Because of delays in the system, women end up having procedures performed outside health facilities by people with no medical training. The majority of bad experiences, or trauma, are as a result of laypeople masquerading as medical personnel and result in harm to women or transgender men, both physically and emotionally. Anti-choice staff and healthcare workers obstruct care or do not use appropriate analgesia. When protocols and guidelines are used and adhered to, abortion is safe and free from dramatisation portrayed in the media.

There are so many cases where women speak about the loss surrounding a miscarriage and the sadness they feel as well as the guilt in terms of not knowing what happened. These feelings will often result in low intimacy, low libido or less enjoyment in sex, further down the line, not because of a sexual health problem but because of unresolved feelings related to the loss of an unborn child. In some instances it's related to women feeling inadequate because they can't conceive or because they continue to have miscarriages. Women who experience spontaneous miscarriages are often given more understanding, leniency and support than those who choose to terminate a pregnancy, or not carry a pregnancy to term.

When giving post-abortion advice I always tell women they need to be on a contraceptive of their choice and if they don't want to be, I give them advice on other methods they can use. Most women are shy and usually ask when they can have sex again and as part of my way of practicing medicine in a very deliberate way, and in the absence of a medical fraternity with a positive sex outlook, I have the conversation around sexual pleasure straight after an abortion. When it comes to women's health, I'm very conscious and intentional when discussing sexual pleasure with them, regardless of what medical diagnosis or condition they have. Waiting another month when they come for their follow-up, may not present itself in the same way to have this conversation.

Unless healthcare providers have these conversations and ask their patients what their thoughts are, they will miss opportunities to share vital information with them. Some women are under so much pressure from their partners pressing them as to when they can have sex, even before the procedure has been done. This pressure, whether it's after childbirth, a hysterectomy, or after treatment for all types of cancer, makes women feel they need to recover quickly just so their partners can start having sex again. Often the coercion to get back to 'normal' is a dominant theme. So many women are in the situation where their only option is to save their marriage by having sex or trying to get their boyfriend not to cheat by having sex. These concepts of having to keep a person who doesn't want to stay with you and who then uses sex as a bargaining chip to stop people cheating, are unhealthy and toxic. Plus, there's also a limit in terms of what we think vaginas have the power to do!

Pregnancy

....

Some of the best times in my career, have been spent listening to women, sociologists, researchers and anthropologists narrate fascinating histories and stories about menstruation, pregnancy and childbirth. A synchronous relationship between the menstrual cycle and the lunar rhythm has been investigated and confirmed by data, laboratory findings, and clinical experience in 826 women. The study I refer to was done in the 1980s and a large proportion of menstruations occurred around the new moon, as compared to other times during the lunar month. Many cultures and families have their own traditions regarding celebratory rites of passage for menarche; the first period. These traditions differ and as cultures evolve, some practices have fallen away. As a young Mosotho, I clearly remember the references made to the moon and tides in relation to my menstrual cycle. In Sesotho, when a woman is on her period, it is said, 'o ya kgweding', meaning 'going to the moon'. A woman in her reproductive years is known as 'o bona matsatsi', with the understanding that if you miss your cycle you are 'o morao', meaning you may be pregnant, or 'o so o le mmeleng' once a pregnancy is confirmed and are thus 'o mo imana', a pregnant woman.

Medical diagnostics has brought with it the accuracy and options of early diagnosis but it wasn't always so. Quickening, the first flutter-like movements made by a foetus, was used as a reference for many as the first confirmatory symptom of a pregnancy. On average, quickening takes place from the 18 to 20-week mark of pregnancy. Some women feel the flutter-like movements from as early as 16 weeks. On the other hand, some women do not even realise they are pregnant! I have examined pregnant women who present at 25 weeks who thought they had gastritis due to the abdominal discomfort and fullness they were experiencing. Even women who have been pregnant before can miss the early symptoms. More and more women arrive at the doctors' rooms after using a home pregnancy test needing confirmation. Many of whom have already had some thoughts regarding the pregnancy. I have learnt that when performing pregnancy tests, it is best to ask, before revealing the results, what kind of reaction the woman would like to hear. By asking this beforehand and providing pregnancy test results with the most appropriate emotion for that woman, relieves many women of performative happiness and lessens any awkwardness that might take over the consulting room. This affirms to the pregnant woman that I respect whatever immediate emotional outcome they experience. Regardless of the circumstances, medical history or decision made regarding the pregnancy, all women must be provided with all the information that enables an informed decision and they must receive care that is dignified, always. The assumption, often based on judgements made about a woman's age, relationship status or social context can make one project expectations about a woman's reaction or as I have experienced, non-reactions coupled with overwhelming shock.

The use of hormonal and non-hormonal contraceptive methods or surgical sterilisation, all of which have a known failure rate, is a personal choice. Some women are not on contraceptives for various reasons; the unbearable and poorly managed side effect profile being one of the most common reasons. To ensure that access to services is timeous, I always include information, when meeting with women about their contraceptive choices, on the signs and symptoms of pregnancy in order to enable women to seek the care they need timeously. If you want to change your current contraceptive method or want to fall pregnant, consult your doctor to discuss the options available and what you can expect. Most commonly used contraceptive methods allow for ovulation soon after you stop using them. For example, after finishing the current box of the pill, fertility should not be affected and in most cases, women usually experience a normal period the next cycle. As with the pill, methods such as the IUD, hormonal arm implant, patch and vaginal ring, fertility is usually restored soon after removal; very often within the same cycle month. However, the injectables and the implant may affect fertility for several months. The return to fertility is so varied that some women have ovulated within a month of stopping the pill while others on the injectable Depo-Provera have a period and ovulation delay of up to two years. The issue of future fertility needs must be discussed as part of the initial consultation about contraception and when circumstances change, as they often do, let your healthcare provider know so they can help you make the decision that is best for you.

Recently, a successful uterus transplant has brought into the spotlight the many ways in which access to modern technology can bring hope to many people who need assisted fertility treatment. Medical advances in the area of fertility management has brought hope and a chance of having children to many who are dealing with various medical, socio-economic, social circumstances. The use of a surrogate to carry a pregnancy and also adoption have remained the main options for those who want a child and to be a parent but for various reasons are unable to biologically do so themselves. Assisted fertilisation has advanced so much in recent years, that the technology is becoming more accessible although the high cost associated still means that only those who are in a financial position to afford it are able to receive assistance that way. The consultation processes also tend to be lengthy depending on the cause that renders one in need of assisted fertility procedures. There are many variations to the technology used in fertility medicine but the concepts are the same.

I have heard every myth in the world regarding how pregnancy actually happens, or what facts make it unlikely to happen, and unfortunately many people believe this incorrect information. Some people falsely believe that having sex standing up will not lead to pregnancy, or that they cannot fall pregnant if they have sex during a period, or when having sex in a pool. While others believe that drinking certain concoctions, such as boiled fizzy beverages, will weaken sperm already ejaculated into the vaginal canal.

A common myth is the belief that the first time someone has sex will not result in pregnancy whereas, in fact, the chances of falling pregnant the first time you have sex is the same as any other time.

There are too many steps to count and even more details to understand about what actually happens when a woman falls pregnant, but I will share as much as is needed for a slightly deeper understanding, but the aim is definitely not to take you through Obstetrics 101! In some cases, in vitro fertilisation, an embryo that is fertilised outside the body, in a fertility lab, is inserted into the uterus for implantation. Using eggs that have been donated is also a possibility for women who are unable to ovulate. In some instances, a woman who is ovulating may also store, through freezing, her own eggs for future use with IVF. Sperm donations are an option when a man cannot produce his own sperm or for those who do not have partners. In this instance, sperm is inserted into the vagina, via a tube, for fertilisation of an ovum that has never been removed.

The biomedical developments available provide more opportunities for sero-discordant couples, meaning where one partner is HIV positive and the other is HIV negative, to have children. When the HIV positive partner's viral load, a numerical number representing the high or low levels of viral copies of HIV in the blood, is undetectable, meaning the viral load is so low that the standard tests used are not sensitive enough to detect the low HIV copies, and when both partners have been treated for any STIs and the HIV negative partner is taking pre-exposure prophylaxis, unprotected sex can allow for conception, as the risk of HIV transmission is greatly decreased by managing all the possible factors in consultation with a healthcare provider. The process of conception involves semen being ejaculated into the vagina during penetrative sex, semen can also travel through the vaginal opening even during ejaculation on the thighs, commonly known as 'thigh sex' where there has not been penetration into the vagina. The sperm travels through the vaginal canal and through the cervix to meet an ovum in the fallopian tubes. The process of conception and fertilisation follows multiple steps and at a microscopic level.

It is worth taking the time to go through the process in order to understand the actual physiology of conception. Look at it as partly myth busting but more importantly, a way to better understand the bodily functions and actions that result in pregnancy.

The uterine contractions experienced during orgasm release the hormone, oxytocin, and the presence of sperm leads to that hormone assisting the sperm in moving through to the fallopian tubes. The mature egg can remain in the fallopian tubes, while making its way into the uterus through the cervix. This process can take up to 24 hours during the most fertile period of a woman's cycle. When the ovum (egg) and sperm are in the same tube at the same time, the sperm penetrates the ovum leading to changes that make it impossible for other sperm to penetrate the mature ovum. The sperm contained in the semen can live up to six days inside the fallopian tube and uterus, and in that time it can still penetrate an ovum if that ovum is released after the sperm arrives in the fallopian tube. After these six days the sperm then dies.

Tip 👍

Pre-ejaculation fluid may contain sperm and the amount of fluid released can be up to 4 millilitres, which means that a woman can fall pregnant even when full ejaculation doesn't occur within the vagina. Although the actual number of sperm in the pre-ejaculate fluid is lower, the concentration and motility of sperm in pre-ejaculation fluid is equivalent to those of ejaculate and this is why the chance of pregnancy remains.

When the sperm cell joins with an egg, this is the process called fertilisation. Once fertilisation occurs, the ball of cells that multiply is called a blastocyst it travels to the uterus three to four days after fertilisation. If the ball of cells attaches to the lining of the uterus this is called implantation and is when pregnancy officially begins. It can take up to two to three weeks after fertilisation for implantation to happen. The mature ovum contains DNA material consisting of 23 chromosomes and the sperm also contains 23 chromosomes. These combine and form a full chromosomal match in the fertilised ovum. After this, a zygote is formed, which starts as a single cell but divides rapidly in the days following fertilisation. The embryo, which becomes the foetus develops from cells on the inside of the zygote and the placenta develops from the cells located on the outside of the zygote.

This sequence is true for a single pregnancy but multiple pregnancies can occur. Identical twins are conceived when one already fertilised egg splits into two separate embryos. Identical contain the same egg and sperm, therefore the same DNA and chromosomes and look exactly alike. Non-identical twins are also called 'fraternal' twins and occur when two separate ova are fertilised by two separate sperm and both fertilised eggs implant in the uterus. They therefore have completely different genetic material. This can happen when the ovaries release more than one ovum, or as a result of certain kinds of assisted fertility treatments such as IVF. People undergoing fertility treatment are often counselled regarding their risks for multiple embryos. Other forms of multiple pregnancies depend on certain odds and no sooner have we heard about the highest number of multiple pregnancies and births, when it seems a record is being broken by someone else.

The hormones released during the menstrual cycle are also responsible for the changes in the lining of the uterus, making it thick and spongy; the favourable condition needed for implantation. A menstrual period occurs if the ovum and sperm do not meet, or a fertilised egg did not result in implantation in the uterus. The thick and spongy lining of the uterus, the endometrium, is then shed as it not required for implantation and moves through the cervix and leaves the body through the vaginal canal and a menstrual period begins.

It is important for a series of hormonal and physical changes that occur in order for implantation to be successful and pregnancy to not be interrupted. Progesterone is the hormone that is released that prevents the lining of the uterus from shedding and this hormone is available for those who may have undergone assisted fertility for various indications or have obstetric history indicating its use in early pregnancy. Progesterone is the main reason why a menstrual bleed does not occur during pregnancy. The sustained level prevents the endometrium from shedding and instead the development of blood vessels occurs, and the thickened endometrium prepare for successful implantation of the fertilised embryo.

It truly is a series of miracles that are required to align for a pregnancy to occur and for those experiencing medical conditions affecting fertility, it can be incredibly frustrating to attempt to control every step of the process.

We have all heard about bizarre pregnancy stories and the TLC show 'I Didn't Know I Was Pregnant' is the most bizarre! I can't get enough of that show and every single time I watch it, my jaw drops in disbelief. It is incredible how extraordinary the body is and how it can accommodate a growing foetus and the harrowing births that many women go through. It is true that there may not be any symptoms at all with early pregnancy and it is not impossible to be pregnant and not know until a few weeks, or even months in some cases, have progressed. Pregnancy does have common signs and symptoms, but not all of these are specific to pregnancy. Some of the symptoms may include a missed period, tender or bigger breasts, nausea and/or vomiting (commonly in the morning although this can happen throughout the day, making the term 'morning sickness' misleading). Other symptoms can include fatigue, poor concentration, feeling bloated, constipation and needing to pass urine more frequently than usual. These symptoms can be similar to those experienced during the premenstrual syndrome (PMS) phase and often are dismissed as such.

There are various ways of calculating how far a woman is in her pregnancy. Gestational age is a medical term used to describe how far along a pregnancy is and this is usually measured in weeks. Gestational age can be counted by several methods; most common is using the start of the last menstrual period which is often abbreviated to LMP. The manner in which pregnancy is measured makes the entire gestation longer than nine months. Any time from approximately 38 to 42 weeks after the last menstrual period is said to be full-term, meaning the gestational period for a mature and fully developed foetus and can turn out to be closer to 10 months than nine months as commonly referred. Full-term refers to completed 37 weeks and preterm refers to a birth less than 27 completed weeks of pregnancy.

For some women, it is not always possible to recall the exact date of their last menstrual period, sometimes the contraceptive method fails and like in the case of injectables, one can ovulate before having a period. Getting medical advice as soon you suspect a pregnancy is possible, is important. This gives you a chance to confirm the pregnancy and consider the options available to you and get information on what to expect and what the next steps could be. Pregnancy is confirmed either by a urine test specific to pregnancy, a blood test that checks for the pregnancy hormone or an ultrasound of the pelvis confirming a presence of a gestational sac or foetus. Only ultrasound measurements of the uterus and the gestational sac or foetus can accurately confirm the gestational period.

Not every pregnancy progresses to full term and even those that do mature to full term do not always end with a healthy baby. Spontaneous miscarriages, induced abortion, all for various reasons, malformations, sometimes for no reason at all, can result in foetal death. In early pregnancy, there are instances where the fertilised ovum, which matures into an embryo, fails to travel down to the uterus or implants in an area unfavourable for foetal growth, such as the fallopian tube, the ovary, cervix or lower abdomen. Many women present to the doctor with symptoms of pregnancy with a positive pregnancy blood or urine test but the embryo is not visualised by the ultrasound scan of the uterus. A sac or an embryo, in some cases, can be visualised in the tubes and this is called an ectopic pregnancy. The main concern with an ectopic pregnancy is that it can cause a rupture and blood loss, leading to shock and sometimes even death. An ectopic pregnancy is a medical emergency and if suspected, medical care must be sought immediately.

The development stages of pregnancy, of which there are three, are called trimesters. The first, second and the third trimesters all have very distinct features of maturation of the foetus as well as accompanying bodily changes for each trimester. Within three weeks, once the embryo is formed, the baby's first nerve cells have already developed. The developing baby is called an embryo from the moment of conception up until the eighth week of pregnancy. Thereafter, until birth, it is called a foetus.

The weight of the foetus throughout the pregnancy is important to guide certain medical interventions and is an indicator to the doctor in terms of overall development. In my experience, many patients are shy or reluctant to discuss the emotional or psychological impact that their pregnancy may be having on them. It is so important that the doctor, nurse or healthcare worker knows how to support you in terms of psychological help. They may refer you to social worker, a counsellor or a psychologist, depending on your needs. I cannot stress enough how important it is to make appointments for regular antenatal check-ups for both medical care and management of any existing medical conditions such as diabetes, hypertension, flare-ups of auto-immune disorders, infectious diseases such as urinary tract infection and HIV. Having regular follow-ups ensures that the growth of the foetus and the overall health of the pregnancy can be monitored.

The labour process is unique and will be different for each person. Pregnancy and labour will also be different from one pregnancy to the next. For some women, labour can be a relatively fast experience, while for others it can take many hours. It is a challenging process on both a physical and emotional level and some women source the services of a doula ('doo-la'; from the Greek meaning 'a female slave'), a professional trained in pregnancy, childbirth, child care and who provides education and support for a woman in labour, or who has recently given birth. The doula is a link between the medical team, the family and woman in labour and assists in helping to hopefully aid in a positive, memorable, and empowering birthing experience. Doulas can also be referred to as labour companions, birth assistants or labour assistants.

More and more women are looking for the services of a doula and the increased interest is a good step. Many women are making an informed decision to include a doula prenatal, during and immediately after labour and for lactation assistance in the weeks after delivery. Doulas are not restricted to birthing and labour and one can opt for a reproductive health doula for support during other procedures such as IVF, abortion and out-of-hospital or home births.

No woman knows how her labour and childbirth will unfold until it actually happens. I was completely overwhelmed, even with all my medical knowledge, and I think I knew too much to be a good patient in the labour ward! I remember asking my mom and my doula, why they never explained how intense the contractions would be and they both responded that they tried! Truthfully, no matter how many books one reads or how many stories you are told, it is only once you are labour that it really sinks in what is happening.

Labour happens in three stages but it may not always be clear when one stage starts and one stage ends. Many women all over the world go through the labour process outside of formal health facilities. Home births are common and, in many communities, access to hospitals or clinics is not guaranteed. Some women may have visiting midwives. The move to de-medicalise births is gaining popularity with more and more women opting to incorporate pilates balls, water births, hypnosis, acupuncture and acupressure into their labour, whether it is in hospital, a clinic or at home. The decision to go through labour outside of a medical facility with no involvement of a nurse or doctor, must be made with an understanding of the risks involved to both the mother and child. Unique birth experiences for low-risk pregnancy and a single non-breech foetus may work out for most people, but there needs to be

157

a plan in place if labour complicates and urgent medical help may be required.

The first stage of labour is when contractions are felt and are regular. These contractions cause the cervix to open or 'dilate', as you will often hear the medical team discuss. The cervix softens, shortens and thins out to allow the foetus to move into the pelvis and birth canal. The first stage of labour is the longest of the three stages and consists of two phases: early labour and active labour. The dilation of the cervix goes from a very small 1 centimetre, a tiny ring, all the way to a 10-centimetre ring, the average size of a melon.

Towards the third trimester of pregnancy, the uterus may start contracting in an unpredictable manner from time to time. These contractions are known as Braxton Hicks. They are usually infrequent and irregular and do not signal labour but are the body's preparation of the uterine muscles for labour. The diagnosis of Braxton Hicks will be made after examination of the foetus, and the cervix.

Preterm labour occurs before 37 completed weeks and unlike Braxton Hicks contractions, these contractions do not slow down; they get longer, stronger, and closer together and they lead to dilatation of the cervix and without intervention to stop the progress, where indicated, active labour will follow. Some risk factors for preterm labour include history of preterm birth, multiple pregnancy (twins, triplets, etc.), abnormalities of the uterus, cervix or placenta, smoking or using drugs while pregnant, high stress levels, certain infections and poor or no antenatal care.

True early labour occurs after 37 completed weeks of gestation and is commonly marked by the expulsion of the mucous plug that blocks the cervix during pregnancy. On average, the length of early labour varies from hours to days and is often shorter in subsequent pregnancies. The start of contractions is the most widely known signal that delivery is impending. The frequency and intensity will gradually increase as active labour begins. The start of labour might also be accompanied by the leakage of amniotic fluid, also commonly referred to as 'the water breaking'. Amniotic fluid is the water that surrounds the foetus inside the placenta and the placenta holds in the fluid during pregnancy. The sac that contains the amniotic fluid is called the amniotic sac. Sometimes the water leakage can be gradual, over a few days, until the major 'water break' during labour and can be followed by vaginal bleeding and passage of mucous discharge.

If this happens away from the facility where you have chosen to deliver, do not delay, get there immediately. It is always recommended to seek medical care when the leakage occurs prematurely, meaning before the pregnancy is term and not in labour, there may be risks of infection to the uterus and foetus, premature birth due to sepsis may lead to bad outcomes.

In early labour, the cervix dilates further at a rate of about one centimetre an hour. If you use a timer to measure the contractions, a pattern will become apparent as the contraction happens at regular intervals of time. They are still mild compared to when in active labour. The contractions feel like a tightening and can last from 30 to 90 seconds. The pain intensifies and this part of labour can last anything from four to eight hours and longer. Childbirth is amongst the most painful experiences known and there are several ways both pharmacologic and non-pharmacologic to assist or be used as treatment. There is no one way of coping with the increasing discomfort and pain; breathing and relaxation techniques, changing of positions, sitting in a water bath and of course the support of family, doula or medical staff can be encouraging.

Unless there is an indication why close monitoring is necessary, taking walks, using a pilates ball and having a gentle massage may help promote comfort during active labour. During early labour, usually hours before active labour, the medical team might recommend drinking small amounts of clear liquids, such as water, ice chips, popsicles or juice, instead of a large, solid meal in case a caesarean section is required later.

In South Africa, approximately 6 out of 10 mothers in the private sector delivered by C-section in 2017; these statistics became evident through reports from medical schemes. These rates are alarmingly high and in some hospitals in Cape Town the rate exceeds 90%, yet the World Health Organisation has historically stated that for any region, the caesarean section rates 'should not be higher than 10 to 15% per country'. Many public health experts warn against these high levels, citing costs, prolonged hospital stays exposing newborns and mothers to hospital-acquired infections as well as post-surgery complications, which could be lessened by having supportive vaginal deliveries, where possible.

Childbirth is one of the most personal experiences and when considering medical interventions and treatment, women consider options to aid in pain relief and take into consideration emotional, psychological, sociologic, and sometimes religious practices or cultural preferences. Pain management options range from oral, intramuscular, intravenous and epidural. The experience of using epidural anaesthesia for labour was reportedly first used in 1909 and since then, vast improvements have been made and today the single bolus epidural has become the most popular method of labour pain management.

Active labour is the stage of labour when the cervix dilates, or opens, from 4 centimetres to 10 centimetres. The contraction may start at the lower back to the abdomen and sometimes the legs may also cramp. Contractions during active labour generally last between 45 to 60 seconds, with three to five minutes of rest in-between.

The time between active labour and the birth of the baby can take longer for those women for whom it is the first time or have had an epidural administered. The baby's head is typically the first part of the body that travels through the cervix and out through the vagina. Sometimes a baby may be breech which means the legs come out first. The vaginal opening has the ability to stretch to allow the baby through.

Different birthing positions are comfortable for different women and therefore should be tried out until you find one that feels best. It is possible that squatting, sitting, kneeling on hands and knees can be comfortable and these positions can also help in delivering the baby.

The monitoring of the progress of labour by medical staff assists in identifying any possible complications that may impact the pregnant woman or foetus. The decision to have an assisted delivery using forceps, for example, or having a caesarean section will often be made at this stage of labour and is influenced by many different factors. The foetus may have a condition that affects the strength of the bones or there may be a bleeding disorder such as haemophilia. The head may not be able to move past the midpoint of the birth canal, or the shoulders or arms present through the birth canal. The size of the foetus or the small size of the pelvis are other factors that may make it hard for the foetus to fit through the pelvis.

The decision to proceed in any one way will be made taking into consideration the possible outcomes and with the guidance of the medical staff. After the baby is born, the delivery of the placenta will follow and mild contractions may continue. During the birth, sometimes the perineum (the area between the vagina and the rectum) tears or is cut, in order to make the birth canal larger, and if necessary this area will be repaired using stitches.

It is not always possible, but the midwife can assist in timing deep breaths and when to push, once the head becomes visible. It may sound strange, but taking breaks for quick short breaths helps the head to

Tips for caring for the perineum:

Place two lubricated fingers (thumb and index fingers) inside the back wall of the vagina and move them from side to side, exerting mild, downward pressure.

Place a warm cloth on the perineum during the active stage of labour.

Use more controlled, gentle and slow pushing during labour to allow time for stretching the perineal tissue.

slowly pass through the vaginal opening, and this will allow the perineum to stretch gently. This is when strong pelvic floor muscles are beneficial to help with strong pushing from the core. Perineal massage is good in the birthing moment and can be performed from 34 weeks onwards. This helps the perineum to become more flexible so it can stretch more easily during labour. Perineal massage may reduce the chances of a natural tear or the need for an episiotomy and it reduces post-delivery perineal pain.

Monitoring will continue well after the delivery. Serena Williams gives a detailed recollection of her time immediately post-partum, when she experienced complications precipitated by her previous medical history of clotting disorders. It can never be stated enough, that should you suspect that you or your newborn baby are unwell, you are uncertain of your condition, or may require medical attention, trust your instincts and let your medical team know.

In Sesotho, the period after delivery is called 'setswetse'. This is when a new mother goes to live with an older woman, either a family member or friend, who then helps with the new baby. The tradition originated when a woman had her first baby and would go and stay with her mother for a few weeks or months. These days some families have developed their own traditions and because of how much families are blended, aunts, older women, younger women and friends often step in to assist the new parents and specifically the new mother. I found this period so incredibly helpful and having my mother take care of me while I took care of my newborn (in reality she took care of us both) was good for my mental and emotional wellbeing. The duration of the length of time 'ya setwetse' takes differs from culture to culture and some families are not as strict as others. Cultures differ and expectations from family and partners are also different. Some families may not choose to have a parent or family member be involved, but I found that having a trusted person close by to offer emotional support, help clean the house, help feed the baby while I bathed, did my hair, or napped (oh my goodness, naps help so much!) is a huge advantage. It is a marvel what the body goes through during pregnancy and the process of birthing and recovery. There are some medical problems that can present after pregnancy or that are related to labour.

After the delivery, it is not uncommon to feel as if the vagina is wider, drier or more swollen than usual. This is normal and will reduce after a few days. Pelvic floor exercises are recommended during and after pregnancy and kegel exercises help tone the vaginal and pelvic floor muscles. Hormonal changes happen soon after delivery and so the lower levels of oestrogen can result in vaginal dryness. Breastfeeding also has an impact on vaginal dryness and the oestrogen levels are lower than for those women who are not breastfeeding. If there are stitches in the perineum, the vulva and vaginal area can be painful, and this should improve as healing takes place in a 6 to 12-week period. It is best to get advice from your doctor or pharmacist before taking any medication for pain especially if you are breastfeeding. There may be vaginal bleeding for some days after vaginal delivery and you will need to take special care of the wound and wash your hands before and after changing the sanitary pads you will need to wear.

There's no right or wrong time to start having sex again after you've had a baby. The standard six-week medical check-up is a good time to discuss any concerns or ask any questions you may have with your doctor or healthcare professional. You more than likely will be feeling tired and not sleeping well (or all that much!) so you won't feel like having sex yet. And that is normal. You do not have to have sex until you feel ready and your vaginal wounds have healed. Should you feel pain or discomfort during sex, you can use a water-based lubricant to decrease any discomfort experienced. You may take time to feel like your old self so if sex hurts, it won't be pleasurable. Don't put pressure on yourself.

It's important to talk about the expectations regarding sex, child-minding, feeding, etc. with your partner, if you have one, during pregnancy, rather than waiting till the baby is born. It is better to be prepared and know that you can depend on open communication, because when one of you is feeling under pressure, it helps being able to deal with things if you are in agreement beforehand.

Common problems experienced by women in the weeks after childbirth:

Some difficulties in managing chronic illnesses such as diabetes, hypertension, thyroid disease, which influence all the metabolic processes in the body.

Excessive vaginal bleeding after delivery

Infections affecting the uterus, bladder and kidneys

Pain in the perineum

Vaginal discharge

Breast problems such as mild swelling, blocked ducts which can progress to an infection called lactation mastitis

Stretch marks, acne, dry skin, hair loss

Haemorrhoids, constipation and urinary incontinence

Post-partum depression

Discomfort during sex

Difficulty regaining pre-pregnancy shape and weight

Section 2

Sexual Pleasure

Why the interest in sex, Dr T?

··

The sexual pleasure revolution as an idea started way before my time and although we only think of sexual pleasure within the context of sexual play or sexual contact with other people, my own personal journey of being conscious of the lack of body positive, sex-positive representation – particularly of women's bodies – was not limited to mainstream media but even as a junior medical student it became clear that even in medicine women's pleasure is not prioritised.

One of the most daunting, but also exciting, aspects of the first year of medical school is human cadaver dissection. I don't know why but even then I was already inquisitive and aware of how little focus was given to female genitalia, specifically the anatomical teachings of the vulva and clitoris, even in that basic introduction to human anatomy. Even during obstetric and gynaecology lectures and tutorials at senior level, the focus of the content was on sexual illness and disease processes and not nearly enough on sexual pleasure.

One would think that, for example, when discussing contraceptive methods with known side effects and sexual dysfunctions such as vaginal dryness, negative impact on libido and the desire for sex and mood changes, women's sexual pleasure and solutions to these issues would be a key area to focus on.

Discussions regarding women's health have been devoid of affirming information surrounding sexual pleasure, and the contrast between what one learns in urology surrounding male sexual dysfunction, biomedical research and solutions around weak erections and early ejaculation, surpassed the equivalent of anything available regarding women's pleasure, even in curricula. Those of us who had developed an interest early on about sexual and reproductive health in relation to women's experiences were let down by our academic textbooks and additional course work that lacked depth and variety of research on these topics.

Even in the speciality of psychiatry, the discussions around sexual dysfunction or mental health that had sexual-related symptomatology, again were lacking in providing young medical professionals with enough of inclusive sexual developmental and normal healthy sexual behaviours, sexual expressions, behaviour, gender and the slant was a very cis-gendered, heteronormative one.

It would be hugely beneficial for young nurses and doctors to qualify with a more refined curriculum and a skill set that will enable them to help patients with gathering their sexual history, manage sexual illness and sexual related issues; the current time demands us as health professionals to be better.

Unfortunately many healthcare professionals, in their own childhood development, have not received comprehensive sexual education and as a result they can perpetuate myths, gender and sexuality biases or discrimination in their patient interactions based on unchallenged prejudices.

Providing personal development for young and old medics alike through a sexual reproductive health and rights framework during undergraduate training and as part of postgraduate continued medical education is vital. Having graduated and being acutely aware of how low sexual pleasure was placed in medicine, as key areas of focus in pharmaceutical development and research, I very quickly developed a bias towards women's health and creating clinical services affirming of women's needs. I was rather drawn to those profiles of gender and sexual minorities because even as a cis-woman (referring to people whose gender identity matches the sex that they were assigned at birth) and as someone who is a woman and was assigned female at birth, I identify as a cisgender woman. I still felt that my sexuality and sexual health were being under-represented.

What then of transgender women waiting to receive affirming healthcare, young people born with HIV as a result of mother to child transmission where the current prevention messaging is altogether missed from their reality, HIV sero-discordant (one person is HIV positive) couples who require assisted fertility procedures in the public sector, women sex workers who require very specific occupational information and screening tests and all of us dealing with the various medical conditions I have discussed in the previous section?

I didn't always know what field of medicine I would specialise in and ultimately end up in, so becoming 'Dr T the Sex Doctor' was the most organic and fulfilling experiences of my life. It was not always clear to me that that would be my speciality as my career seemed to take a lot of time to define itself in terms of what it was about sexual and reproductive health that was important to me. I felt I could have the most impact in the area of sexual pleasure, particularly women's sexual pleasure, throughout our different reproductive cycles. Meeting women, hearing about their experiences, thoughts, feelings, how we as women experience our bodies through menopause, menstruation and through sexual violence and trauma and what that would look like, not just for women in general but for South African women, became my focus.

South Africa has very specific circumstances in that not only was there previous legislative violence that came with apartheid but also healthcare was not designed for black women. We are also living in a country where the extremely high levels of sexual violence, harassment and rape mean that not only do most of us know someone who has been violated in some way, but many of us carry with us experiences that we are not always sure of in terms of what they actually 'mean'. It was only once I started doing work on radio, in print and hosting sex toy parties, when I realised a lot of what I knew to be true for myself was affirmed by other women's experiences. Some of the issues included consensual sex within long-term relationships, such as marriage, or couples struggling with fertility treatment, where for them sex almost feels like a chore and then starts to mean a different thing to them as a couple.

As a young doctor, often young people – my peers – would ask me very personal questions about their own journeys and I think this is because there is an assumption that I am less judgemental because of my closeness in age. Because we had had similar experiences, more and more people would confide in me, even if they didn't know me. This highlighted for me the need for knowledge and help and pushed me to keep doing what I was doing. If people find you naturally receptive and can look at you and feel you are someone who can help them with some of the most deepest and most intimate experiences of their lives, that's when I realised I could have a meaningful impact. There has to be a need based on young people coming to me with the same questions surrounding sex, sexuality, relationships, break-ups and issues around safe terminations and HIV.

So as much as I too was discovering 'Dr T the Sex Doctor' through my interactions with young people at local clinics, I found myself reading more, broadening my understanding and interrogating my own sexuality and fluidity and what it meant for me to be doing this work and how much it means for my own personal experience.

Often when you have deep meaningful conversations with patients they tend to become less of the typical doctor/patient conversations, and often you are challenged in ways you aren't always ready for. In addition, I did not always know or have all the answers so I became a student of my patients. Also because of my medical expertise we were both 'giving and taking' within the consultations. There was also something very meaningful in not having time constraints when consulting and people valued that I was taking them seriously when they mentioned a sexual health or sexual pleasure-related issue.

My extended reading had started to include menopause, the contraceptive pill and the adverse effects that come with it so I had started developing a way of consulting that offered people information without them asking. If I heard someone was on a contraceptive, I would then offer them information about lubricants, the link to contraception and how they could expect certain side effects with different contraceptives.

What often caught me off guard was how correct my intuition had been as a young medical professional, not being given any of the information and even finding the necessary information was difficult, so I knew then that my feelings of inadequacy were valid. Often I would need to refer and read and find information and find other doctors and writers who had different ways of practising medicine and reproductive health and that has really determined a large part of my career path and the spaces that I currently find myself in.

Today, a lot of the focus is around the sexual revolution but also about what it means for us in different locations we inhabit geographically and the spaces we take up, the demographics and types of illness that people in different countries experience.

In South Africa, the issues of breast and cervical cancer and HIV are the most worrisome in terms of new infections. Also, how we talk about things related to sex, about HIV, sex after a spinal injury, sex after sexual assault, etc. It has been an experience of growth for me not only as a doctor but personally and because I have allowed myself to take and be a part of a journey and immerse myself within the experiences and the stories. Not only do I open myself up to new experiences from very different people, from all walks of life and of all ages, they feel heard and know I take them seriously. Many patients I see often have the same history. Whether its how many doctors they've consulted and none of them seem to be able to help, or no one takes them seriously regarding vaginal dryness or how someone can be raped and still want to enjoy sexual pleasure, these are recurring themes and issues. I am walking that road with all my patients who come in for therapy and sexual health-related consultations and feel like they have all chosen me to walk this path with them. And for that, I'm lucky.

Sexual consent

Consent for any sexual contact or act is when the people involved in that specific contact or act agree to take part in it; whether it's kissing or touching, oral sex or vaginal sex, and of course using body parts and other objects, such as toys, as part of the sexual contact or act that is being agreed upon.

It's always fascinating to me, especially because of the travelling and the work that I do in terms of sexual pleasure and the sexual pleasure revolution, that around the world there are so many laws that govern sexual contact and consent. Yet the age limits are very different.

South Africa has a very specific Sexual Offences Act, which obviously supplements the Constitution and the right to dignity and freedom to choose. It's particularly important to take into consideration the legal framework, as one of the problems from the previous laws surrounding this is that children would be criminalised for being peers in the same age group engaging in sexual activities or exploring themselves sexually; whether that's kissing or full-on sexual contact.

What's important is how do we have the discussion of sexual pleasure within this violent world and society we're living in, and what does consent then look like in that environment? I've had a lot of women – survivors of sexual violence – who, for many years, can't have sex in the way that they want to. Whether that is as a result of anxiety or a previous trauma, some women are not even aware that their lack of desire for sex is directly linked to a violation that might have happened to them before.

In some cases, when talking to older people, some of them need to 'relearn' how to have healthy sex again. These conversations would be impossible without actually talking about consent and what went 'wrong'. But it is also vital for engaging in future healthy sex interactions.

South Africa is rife with the blesser/blessee relationships, which frankly, for me, stigmatises women and to exceptionalise it is something I struggle with. It is as if millennials have come up with 'new' promiscuous ways when, in all honesty, this is no new phenomenon. All the societies of the world have been designed in such a way that women have always had less power, less economical resources. Women are still the ones employed in low-paying jobs and so there has always been a dominance of men with power and resources. Women were (and in many, many cases still are) at some point in their lives, dependent on men and money.

This is the reason I rather focus on what the drivers and pressures are that young women are facing that make them unable to negotiate safer sex with whoever they are having sex with. Everyone looks at the blesser/blessee in terms of the transactional sex and of course the HIV transmission but no one talks about the fact that many young women are in relationships with men of their own age and from their peer group and those young women are suffering physical violence and death in some instances. There is a misconception that if you don't go out with someone who is older than you and just stick to your peers, you'll be fine. The research shows that you won't be fine.

The issue of healthy sex lives and of negotiating healthy sex is a universal thing, not an age thing. Of course there could be power dynamics with your peers that you will have to overcome but we know things are still very much skewed where women have less power. There are laws that govern who can give consent and who can't give consent and when consent can happen. It needs to be completely clear between the people involved and consent has to be actively sought. In no world does, 'I took you out for dinner' or 'we've been chatting on WhatsApp' or 'you've sent me a nude' or 'you've been sexting me' means there is any consent to having sex.

Things such as relationship status do not constitute consent forever. Some women are married but it doesn't mean that because they are married they have given consent perpetually to have sex within their marriage. The issue of consent and sexual violation is so often looked at only with people who are not married or are single but the issue of marital rape is a huge problem that is not talked about. So many women who are married are unable to share because there is this idea that married women have a chore and duty to make sure that their partner has sex. There is a saying that you need to give your husband or partner sex so that they don't go and look elsewhere. There is extreme anxiety and a burden on women that if they do say no to having sex with their husband, then if the husband chooses to have sex with someone else, she can't say anything.

The people involved in sexual experimentation, contact, or act must be of a legal age and have the mental ability and capacity to understand and respond. Some people are mentally unable to fully understand what consent means perhaps because of a medical reason or developmental issue. Saying that a child, a minor, has 'given consent' is a crime. Their age limits them from having the cognitive ability to understand what it is that you want to do to them. Often people say the child or the young person said it's 'fine', or they didn't scream and/or say 'no'.

Consent for sexual contact consists of more than a 'yes' or a 'no'. It must involve the details of condom use, what kind of sexual positions you'll be doing and what body parts are involved. Often people think when they say 'let's have sex' they just have sex, but often the partici- pants haven't discussed the actual details of the sex. It's not just a yes or a no. What about how do you want it? How will I know when you've had enough?

There's this obsession with a man's erection and ejaculation, in that sex starts with his erection and ends with ejaculation. There is not much else in-between that is affirming for women or for the person receiving that penis. We should get to a point where people are not shy to explain and say what it is that they want as part of that initial consent of 'do you want to have sex or not'. You have to ask; whether it's kissing or hugging, oral sex or foreplay, if you haven't asked you don't have consent.

People say it's boring when you're in a relationship with someone because you know each other and you know what they like but there is a place for learning each other's language and body language and it has to be a deliberate step. You have to talk about the fact that when I say I want to have sex I may not say it out loud or I might start touching you or rubbing your ear. Whatever that detail is, it cannot just be assumed that when you touched her vagina and it was wet, it meant she wanted to have sex. It does not work that way.

There is a certain way you can have these discussions with your partner. It doesn't always have to be through words but you need to have a predetermined discussion. When it comes to kink or fetishes, consent around this is vital. If someone is blindfolded or they have a sock in their mouth and can't speak, or their hands are tied up, what does consent look like in that situation? The blindfold is covering the person's eyes and a sock prevents the person from being able to say 'no', so how are boundaries put in place in this instance?

The point is that consent is about more than just whether you want to have sex or not. No is enough, even though there so often is pressure to explain why. It's that pressure that makes people hesitant to say no out loud and then rather avoid the issue or pretend they didn't hear. One of the issues I hear all the time from young people is that they can't say no when they don't want to have sex because they think that will lead to a break-up of their relationship.

When we say people must expect their consent to be respected, we need to look at it from both sides. If you are the one asking for consent and someone says no, what are your responsibilities? Often we burden the people from whom consent is being sought but we never give the responsibility to the person who has asked for the consent, and say that when someone has said no or yes, what does it mean? I once had a patient who said she knew that she should be saying no when she didn't want to have sex but couldn't, because her partner would question her and accuse her of cheating and ask who else she had been sleeping with and accusing her of not 'loving me any more'.

The issue of pressuring people, I suppose, works on the issue of dominance. People think that if you say no, you actually mean yes and they must then pursue you harder or it means you are playing hard to get. When I was growing up, boys asked girls to go out with them and even after saying you did not want to go out with them, they would try twist our arms by carrying our bags and try various tactics to try pressurise us into agreeing. They would sometimes ask if it was because they didn't have a car, or for some other superficial reason and we would be made to feel guilty by them, highlighting any deficiencies they think they had that were making us say no. Burdening someone by making them feel, 'I'm a bad person for saying no, I'm hurting this person by making them feel like they're not good enough' are manipulative tricks and threats of violence that become all too real.

Many married women or those in long-term partnerships, often describe the force or threat of physical violence that can accompany their partners' requests for sex. For example, threatening to throw her out of the house at 2 am or the constant threat of 'if you don't oblige I will do something to hurt you'.

Today, with the proliferation of nude images and sexting, a lot of threats revolve around men threatening to expose videos or post nude images of their partners on social media. This is revenge porn and the dark side of what technology can do. But unfortunately what people still don't understand, in terms of technology and consent and sex, is how, in some spaces, it can be empowering to make use of technology to enhance sexual pleasure.

When I run workshops for young people about sexual pleasure and sexual health, I always give them the example that there is no 'safe' place to find guidance on how to take a nude in such a way that if someone violates your trust and shares or posts it on the internet tomorrow it won't link to you. What happens when someone invites you to their place and says you must start kissing or having sex, are you thinking

176

about whether or not they may be secretly recording? There is nowhere to go in the world that doesn't have smartphones or access to devices that can record or film.

We need to find the balance between not scaring young people off, but at the same time sharing the real consequences of sexting and sending video clips and nudes in a way that if someone shares them without your consent how the situation can be managed. Basic but essential tips include taking the photo without your face in it, making sure the mirror isn't showing your reflection and deactivating anything that could lead people to physically locating you at your home address or from a landmark. It's also important to remember to not include the date the photo was taken or show any identifying marks such as piercings, tattoos, birthmark, scars.

The approach that needs to be taken is around erotic intelligence; cyber erotic intelligence. Back in the sixties, porn was shot by production companies on VHS cassettes but soon camcorders became available and people could buy their own handheld cameras and this completely blew up the porn industry. All of a sudden, individuals became producers of pornography. Today, young children have access to smartphones, data, the ability to photoshop and edit, making it so, so important to have the discussion around cyber erotic intelligence. There have been a lot of cases in South Africa where young people have been exposed and the trauma that goes with that can be incredibly traumatic and in some cases even lead to suicide. This mostly happens to young girls and women, and so the issue of consent needs to be thought about and discussed far beyond a 'yes' or 'no' at the beginning of the encounter.

I also feel so strongly about the fact that when someone gives you gifts, takes you on a holiday, or is nice to you, and happens to perhaps be your parent's friend/cousin/uncle, no one has the right to demand sexual favours from you. Even in the workplace, a lot of people are expected to perform sexual favours to get a promotion or to secure a job.

Consent as a whole is the overarching issue but each sexual pleasure 'theme' in this section has certain aspects that will speak to consent about that specific issue and how to communicate with your partner about having, for example, anal sex and the issues and feelings around that.

Medical conditions such as fibroids, pelvic pain, endometriosis, etc., all present various difficulties when it comes to having sex and having that discussion is all part of consent. Issues of grief, such as how do you move on after your partner has passed away and are feeling inquisitive again, are all areas that need to be discussed. How does it look for you internally to give yourself that permission to be experimental again?

Consent is mandatory, it's not sexy. Our society is conflating very basic human rights requirements, such as consent, HIV testing, STI treatment and turning it into something playful and sexy. What does sexy look like? Do I need to be a sultry, leopard-print lingerie-wearing goddess to be, and feel, sexy? When do I become sexy in the process of consent or getting an HIV test?

Consent is compulsory and it *always* matters, regardless of the relationship status, irrespective of whether you've had sex with that person before and regardless of how adventurous you have been in the past. Consent always matters and the details of that consent always matter. It has to be clear for everyone involved what the agreement is. People do have sex with multiple partners so the time has to be taken to get consent from each person involved. And consent has to be sought about using sex toys. There is no sexual pleasure without consent.

When it comes to sexual violence, when someone keeps quiet, that doesn't necessarily mean it's a yes. The absence of a 'no' is not a 'yes'. A 'no' can present itself in many different ways where some people are triggered and freeze and some people are just too scared to say anything.

Consent needs to be given enthusiastically, in an affirming way without pressure or coercion and on an ongoing basis, even if during sex you decide to try something new or different, even when things are flowing and sparks flying, it's important to keep talking and being attentive to the feedback given. If you're silent during sex how are you going to tell your partner to go deeper or harder or slower?!

People feel so shy to talk during sex, which seems strange for me personally. I think because I hear so many stories during therapy sessions, the shyness of women, especially, talking during sex and saying what feels good for them, is often what they get judged on. They are called 'sluts', because how do they know what feels good and why do they want to change the position or who did they try it with before? The ability for women to feel pleasure and be completely immersed in that sexual experience is often limited by the fact that they already know they will be judged for asking for sex in a certain way or position.

The work of the pleasure revolution is important, and it wouldn't be complete without talking about the pressure, the societal ways and views of what women are entitled to and what they do not have to accept. But that's maybe for the next book! Right now we are going to talk about all things pleasurable but it was important to set the context of consent because there is no fun without consent.

The Big O

....

The orgasm. For some people it's elusive while others have experienced some mind-numbing, toe-curling explosive and all the other amazing ways people describe their orgasms. I think faking an orgasm is very much like scoring your own goal. Most people will fake an orgasm during penetrative sex, but it does also happen during oral sex, while having phone sex and any other times where people feel pressure to make their partner feel validated. People think only women can fake orgasm but men, or at least those with penises, can also fake an orgasm. Often if a person realises, or finds out the other person is faking an orgasm, they may feel cheated, lied to or hurt, incorrectly believing they had been pleasuring you.

People give various reasons for faking orgasms; one being that they want to avoid hurting their partner's feelings. Others want their partner to think they're good in bed while some just want the sex to end. Because sex is assumed to end with orgasm people don't feel comfortable to say they've had enough and would rather just talk instead. Research in the *Journal of Sex Research* suggests that the sexual script that says women should have orgasms before men, and that men are responsible for women's orgasms, can lead to a very rigid overall experience. It's worthwhile to really interrogate our own predetermined sexual script and how that then puts pressure on your sexual partner. For example, I'm having sex but I don't necessarily care to have an orgasm, but if you are my partner and you are judging my sexual fulfilment based on an orgasm, it means there is pressure to fulfil your idea of what pleasure means to me as your partner.

When people's expectations and their sexual pleasure or enjoyment are not matching up, chances are higher that someone will fake something at some point. Especially if you're not talking to each other and describing what feels good, whether that be to go deeper, faster, slower, harder. Talking to each other during sex can be the most intimate way of communicating and a way to get rid of the 'scripts'. This also helps set the tone and can, for those with bad memories of previous experiences, give you a chance to get the sex you want.

There are many factors that play into achieving an orgasm. The issue of emotional readiness is underestimated on the one hand and over-exceptionalised in another. There is a level of emotional maturity and cognition required for sex, hence we have important things such as the age of consent and they are nuanced and take into account mental capacity as well. For some people raised in very religious homes where the views around sex are extremely conservative, their childhood is filled with fear-driven and dominating themes that sex is sinful and they therefore, even as adults, find it hard to switch off the gospel from the megaphone and find it difficult to give themselves permission to enjoy sex because for them sex carries negative connotations.

Women often perform acts that are meant to symbolise love and desire for love attachments in order to minimise being shamed for flirting, being sexually expressive and being involved in sexual play. These performances (and I call them that because without the judgement, many women wouldn't be concerned about what people think of them) are usually done to prove they are not cheap, slutty or loose. Yet men are given more leeway regarding casual sex, such as one-night stands, without the sustained judgement.

Sexual trauma is another factor that can make it very difficult for someone to achieve an orgasm. Issues of negative body image, feelings about your partner, feelings about yourself, are all anxieties that can add up and make orgasm a major issue for some people. For many people – specifically women – they often don't have a problem having an orgasm when they're masturbating and will have sex with their partner, perhaps fake an orgasm and then masturbate on their own because they know they will be able to have an orgasm. Some women don't mind not having an orgasm but enjoy the actual sex. My advice is, your hands are free, so stimulate your clitoris or vulva in a way that can enhance and increase your chances of achieving an orgasm during sex, if that's something that is important to you.

Women can also feel more relaxed with their partner if they have some self-play time too. Again, the scriptedness of how sex should happen puts pressure on women so if they have as much time as they need, because there's no risk of a man losing his erection, indulge in self-play. It can only add to your sexual experiences with your partner. Vibrators, sexual stimulation toys, lubricants, can all be helpful in exploring your body. There is a misconception surrounding lubricants that I feel I need to mention, in that lube should be normalised as something to use during sex and not something you should wait to use if you feel you are having problems becoming aroused. During a normal menstrual cycle, there are variations on the amount of lubrication you will naturally produce so using lube when having sex only enhances the experience.

The longer you are in the pre-orgasmic zone, that is, lingering longer in sexual play and incorporating lube and sex toys, the greater the chance of achieving an orgasm and the more intense it will be. You need to know what makes you aroused. What does it feel like when I'm at my maximum point of arousal? You may use a certain kind of fantasy to get you there. Perhaps relaxation techniques, erotic literature or movies help you get in that zone. Figure out what it is that works for you. Pay attention to that path of arousal. Practice it and share it with your partner.

During an orgasm there's the peak; first the foreplay, then the sex – the thrusting – and there the peak is followed by a plateau. The intensity is in that peak, and there will still be some intensity after the peak so it's important to enjoy that moment too and not just roll over and pass out!

There is also always the possibility of getting intimate again, and, yes, there is lots you can do with a flaccid penis after ejaculation; you don't always need an erect penis to have fun. If you don't have an orgasm you can still carry on and that analogy of sex starting with an erection and ending with an ejaculation isn't right, there is still more you can do after that – at least for a few more minutes. Clitoral stimulation is something you can do because that doesn't require penetration and neither does G-spot stimulation. There are various positions you can try and the use

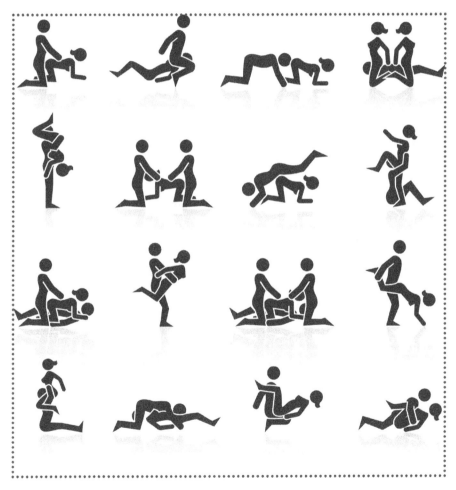

Sexual positions

of fingers or toys can elevate a perhaps mediocre sexual experience into an intense, orgasmic experience.

Some women have orgasmic dysfunction and have extreme difficulty achieving an orgasm during sex or masturbation. This is not exclusive to a partner and can be called generalised orgasmic disorder because they are able to have an orgasm on their own but not with someone. Women who never experienced an orgasm have a condition called primary anorgasmia. However, if a woman has difficulty reaching an orgasm even if she has experienced one before, it is called secondary anorgasmia. The most common type of orgasmic dysfunction is called situational orgasmic dysfunction and occurs when a women can only have an orgasm in certain situations or with certain kinds of stimulation. Some people can only have an orgasm during oral sex, or while masturbating, and that is known as situational anorgasmia. If someone is able can give themselves an orgasm but can't have one with a partner this is also situational anorgasmia. Inability to achieve orgasm, under any circumstance, even when you are highly aroused and sexual stimulation is sufficient is called general anorgasmia.

The symptom of orgasmic disorder is defined as 'the lack of or delay in sexual climax (orgasm) even though sexual stimulation is sufficient and the woman is sexually aroused mentally and emotionally'. Usually a woman notices this lack or delay over a period of time. Not having an orgasm once or twice is not usually an indication of a bigger problem, as a disorder is a pattern where despite becoming aroused, a woman doesn't achieve an orgasm. In this instance, assistance should be sought.

Sometimes there may be an underlying medical problem or a side effect of medication that's causing you to have orgasmic issues. In this case it's wise to consult your health provider and see if they can substitute your medication or hormonal therapy. Individual and couple counselling can also help in this regard because once you are feeling anxious and already have negative feelings about sex you may not be able to 'self-help', in which case it's advisable to get help as an individual or as a couple.

It's normal to not have an orgasm every time you have sex and depending on what you desire, you may be satisfied with a few orgasms every now and then. Some women may have an orgasm and still find it unsatisfying while others take longer than normal to reach an orgasm and this can lead to frustration, and the anxiety then starts settling in as a result. If you have any relationship stressors, they may contribute to your inability to have an orgasm.

Conservative cultural belief systems and virginity pacts or purity pledges can affect a woman's relationship and sex life as a whole, in the long term, as well as possibly hampering her ability to fully immerse herself in the sexual experience, have an orgasm and experience sexual pleasure. Sometimes it's worthwhile spending time on understanding your own value system and beliefs about your own sexual experiences and your body.

I've had the privilege of listening to many people talk about their ideas of sex, sexual satisfaction, values, fears and experiences about sex. A few years back I was on the air on KayaFM's sexual health feature that we had every Thursday. After what was meant to be a once-off baby-making discussion, eventually turned into a weekly slot due to the overwhelmingly positive response we received. The feedback from the listeners, mostly from young black women, was that they had never had a space where they were able to talk about their bodies and really embrace and 'own' their sexual experiences.

That specific day we had an open line, where listeners could set their own agenda and ask anything, We'd usually get calls about topics ranging from relationship advice, a bit of health and then the usual from men like, 'is my penis long enough?' 'can I have more rounds in one night?' 'what can I use to make it longer or bigger?' When women phoned in it was usually about a previous bad experience – whether it was trauma or just bad sex – or a medical issue like their contraceptive/antidepressants affecting their sex drive. Some questions were about kids and others that they were just exhausted. Others asked about how to have the best sex life ever. It was a range.

You never know what you are going to get so I was always ready for anything, and that is what deepened my love for sexual health. I read journals, I was keeping up with the World Association of Sexual Health, and I wanted to broaden the conversation because anyone can Google the effects of contraceptives but there is a way you can bring it into a South African context.

That day, the topic we ended up talking about was labial elongation. Listeners were interested in this because it is something practiced in Southern Africa and often associated, specifically, with the Basotho women. Young girls or women elongate their labia over time, not in terms of genital modification (which for some people has a negative connotation) but in terms of sexual enhancement. The Basotho women know that the labia consists of smooth muscle which contracts. Because the labia is part of the vulva, during sexual penetration or stimulation you will increase your chances of having an orgasm because the clitoris itself extends into the labia. So, if you stretch the labia or elongate them, you almost increase the surface area of where it's possible to have an orgasm when stimulated. The more the area of erogenous zones, the higher your chances are of having an orgasm. I had a discussion with my mom around labial elongation and when I asked her who decides whether a woman must do it or not, she responded that a woman decides for herself, when she is older, but to remember that once the labia are elongated, they can't be made to go back to how they were. So if labial elongation is something you might be interested in, give it some careful thought.

After the discussion that day, we had a caller phone in by the name of Lebo. Her query was pretty 'tame' in that she asked me to explain to her where her G-spot was. I had been speaking about the G-spot before her call came in as it is a topic that comes up all the time so I starting explaining to her in a technical and medical way using anatomy and physiology. I told her the G-spot is elusive for many people but you can actually find it so I literally started giving her the 'directions'. If you are lying flat on your back imagine a line leading down from the belly button to the pubic hair. You'll feel the pubic bone and if you move further south you will then feel some fat cushioning and the pubic area, that's your mons pubis. Further down from that is where you'll find the actual vulva starts. It's meaty, the outer lips are there and under the hood, right in the middle will be your clitoris. You can stay there and tingle and play around a bit and get going to find the G-spot.

I always push things to the edge, so I used religious references and said to her that if she opened and spread the inner lips, the labia minora, it would be like opening a Bible. I was extremely mindful that while Lebo was the one that was calling, there may have been other people listening who also didn't know where their G-spot is, so I was very technical and quite graphic in my descriptions. In my mind I was a medic explaining physiology to someone and I wasn't really paying attention to what was coming through on the other side of the phone, but she was really paying attention so I kept going because she wasn't interrupting me at any point.

I then told her to move further down to the vaginal opening and insert her finger about a centimetre and a half into the vagina. I told her to really feel as so often women are either inserting a tampon or washing and not much else and are not familiar with what their vagina actually feels like. I often use the analogy of getting into a driveway and then just sitting. Ask yourself, 'What does it feel like?' So often sensuality and arousal is about taking time, getting your brain to feel what you're feeling and getting rid of any negative feedback and the noise inside your head. This is what encourages the sexuality and the spark. I then carried on speaking about lubricant and masturbation and how helpful it can be.

By this point I realised that Lebo was doing exactly what I was explaining and while she wasn't just taking it all in, she was actually exploring as I spoke! I wasn't at all prepared for that but if that was where we're going, then that was where we were going!

I had been on the show for about three years at that time and the team had developed a certain language and code amongst ourselves;

if you had an orgasm or sexual climax we would say that person was going to Polokwane! So by this point we knew Lebo's destination and I could see the host had an expression of glee on her face! We then cut to an ad break and the silence on the phone was a certain kind of quiet that wasn't 'empty air' and so I asked Lebo what she was doing. Without any hesitation she responded, 'Exactly what you've been telling me to'. We didn't want to put Lebo off and make any exclamation but we were both very excited.

I realised I needed to get consent from her to carry on but we she was doing it and being live radio we couldn't do much. She confirmed she was happy to carrying on exploring. This was a new experience for me too as I had never given someone step-by-step instructions on how to have an orgasm. Lebo sounded quite confident and comfortable and said we should carry on and see where it took us.

So we go back live after the ad break and I told the listeners what was happening, that Lebo was live, so if anyone felt uncomfortable now would be a good time to stop listening as I was going to carry on with the instructions and see how far it would take us. I told Lebo to think of the fabric, corduroy, as that is what it feels like inside the vagina around the G-spot area. The trick is to stimulate it, and it's going to feel good, but there's a point where you are going to feel almost uncomfortable and an intensity like you want to pee. But you have to stimulate and enjoy beyond that point because that's actually where the orgasm and the magic lies – it's after that feeling of 'oh my gosh'.

And as I said this, Lebo let out the deepest moan and groan, and then a huge sigh. She had a whole orgasm live on radio on a Thursday night. In hindsight, I think we were all far too brave! This was stuff you couldn't script!

Lebo taught me so much. First of all, she didn't know me, she knew my voice and knew *of* me but she trusted me and what I was saying so much, that she felt comfortable enough to try it right there and then. This made me wonder how transformative it would be if that level of trust and clarity was present between people who were actually looking at each other, having those experiences together. How much deeper and organically beautiful that experience would be for them.

The phone lines crashed after Lebo had her orgasm! All was quiet and we all looked at each other, taken aback and still questioning whether it had actually happened! Because KayaFM is an independent station, there was just that much more we could do to push the envelope a little bit. I still don't know if anyone ever complained about that show but because we always had an 'explicit' jingle disclaimer at the beginning of the show, we were covered.

On another show not long thereafter we got a call from a man saying he needed help. He was a newly married man and both he and his wife were very religious and had never had sex. They were both virgins and he had no idea what to do, where to go and how to start. In a very similar way to Lebo, I knew he needed my technical and practical advice so I told him that if his wife was there with him, to look at the line leading down from her belly button and follow the path to the Garden of Eden! I think I was feeling quite smug after Lebo's call! He asked if he could try it and I encouraged him to do so and reminded listeners to be gentle and kind lovers. That couple went and did their exploring and then sent a follow-up email confirming all my tips had worked.

Often people think that when you talk about sex there is a sleaziness to it or a dirty way to make it sound raunchy or sexy but that day I was just being literal and technical about the information, using anatomy and 'landmarks', and yet we all had fun! Sex and sexual pleasure isn't just for sex kittens, we are all sex kittens in our own right, just find the kitten that works for you.

The point is they didn't know me, but while using very medical and sterile terminology, we were able to make that magic. Imagine then how empowering it would be to be able explain to your partner what it is that you want. People still reference Lebo or the couple when they see me today, three years later, and about what that show meant to them and I always use those two stories to drive home the message of clarity. Say what it is that you want, and it doesn't have to be raunchy or naughty or dirty, literally just say what you need to get out of the experience.

Another caller that was memorable for me on that show, was when a woman phoned in and said she was sitting in a taxi on her way home. Because the taxi's shock absorbers were worn out, every time they went over a speed bump she felt vibrations in her pelvic area. Being in the seated position, in an overcrowded taxi, she was so hot and flustered she thought it was probably because everyone was so squashed together. She then said that one last bump the taxi took caused her to have such an intense feeling in her vulva that she had an orgasm. She literally cried out and then had to silence herself the rest of the way. She shared her story with us as we had been talking about why women have silent orgasms and because she had such an intense experience of one she wanted to share it with us.

So, in closing, remember, orgasms can happen in the most exciting of places and ways, there is no script and your body will do what it wants. And to this day, every time I see a taxi, I always wonder how good its shock absorbers are.

Sexual fantasy

During the many radio interviews and the frequent times I give comment for print interviews, I am often asked to comment on whether sexual fantasies are a form of cheating. I always have to emphasise that sexual fantasies are part of normal sexual expression and not in any way peculiar. In fact, sex starts in the brain and fantasies happen in the brain. You colour in and fill in the details of the fantasy from your imagination. If you can fantasise and imagine the sexual experiences you want to have, where and with whom, fantasising is a good resource for private experimentation.

You may be inquisitive within the same sexual orientation or want to explore other areas such as kink, submissive/dominant role play or use sex toys. It can take a while for people to be erotically free in their own minds, to talk 'dirty' to themselves or masturbate. Across the world, in many cultures and religious dogma, sex continues to be the subject of judgemental undertones and moralistic and oppressive views creating and deepening the taboos, myths and fear associated with pleasure and sexuality in general. These views and prejudice can make it difficult for some people and the journey to being sexually liberated can be protracted.

Sexual fantasies are common and many people do partake in them whether it's during partner arousal or sex itself. Some people can fantasise about the person they are currently with or the main character in their fantasy may be someone other than the person they are having sex with. This often makes people feel like they are being dishonest or cheating. One of the most common things women experience is that while they are having sex with their partner they are fantasising about another woman or the subject of their fantasy is something they would ordinarily not find arousing, but within the sexual act it turns them on. This is sometimes how interest in kink or role playing can start.

Fantasies can be very different and diverse; some can be outright bizarre and erotically imaginative; from the location, what is being done to the people involved, and they can be linked to a person's past experiences or future desires. A fantasy can be a reflection of current needs and because they are so deeply personal they provide an insight of sorts into the individual's private world of erotic imagination.

Some people have a consistent theme of what their fantasies look or sound like while others may add detail every time. Some people may start having a fantasy with self-pleasure and masturbation and their fantasy then takes on a different scenario where other people get involved. This can sometimes be influenced by real-life experiences. It's almost like having a crush on someone; you know the probability of a real-life sexual experience is low, yet you may form a personal and private imaginative erotic experience.

Some people's fantasies might revolve around role playing where a person fantasises about their partner wearing a certain type of uniform. (*Think navy officer, ladies!*) Fantasies depend on the person and the varieties are far ranging. Themes such as domination and submission, being kinky, using latex catsuits, being strapped up and bonded, having a tie or cloth applied over your eyes to restrict your visual stimulation, or having your hands tied up, are all fairly common fantasies. They can involve strangers or an ex-lover, celebrity or film star.

Sometimes people fantasise about being watched by others and people's sexual fantasies will be informed by their views on sex and how comfortable they feel in their own body. Often you will find that as you get older, your fantasies might change. When your feelings of your own self-exploration reaches certain stages, so too will your fantasies change. It is important to realise that sexual fantasies do form an important part of sexual play and it is normal to fantasise.

Sometimes the fantasy would not work in real life – because maybe it involves your boss – so the main thing is to realise that there is a level of control and responsibility that you should hold because you do not want to be fantasising about coercive behaviour or inappropriate subjects.

The scenarios that people respond to or find to be an aphrodisiac carry with them a responsibility such as role-playing fantasies that do not encroach on other people's rights and dignity. Sexual fantasies should be in line with that. Some people are happy not to have their sexual fantasies lived out in real life and they may use their sexual fantasy as a secondary place, a sort of a secret world they have created. People can feel guilty or anxious because of the content of their fantasies and this might be an issue due to not having been introduced to sexual talk in your relationship to make it okay for people to have these fantasies outside of long-term partnerships. Often married couples feel guilty about having fantasies outside of their relationship.

Sexual fantasising can be useful, especially early on in relationships when couples are still trying to get to know each other. Letting someone new share in your wildest fantasies can help them understand what it is you may want to do as well as help them manage their own expectations. No one should feel strange if they don't partake in their partner's sexual fantasy or in imagery. People need to know that how they approach or respond to aphrodisiac or erotic material, is okay.

Often when people have fantasies of certain scenarios there can be a tendency to try to force a partner to enact those fantasies. But it is so important to make sure that your fantasy is shared by your partner and not presume they automatically share it.

The only way you know how far your partner will be willing to go along with your fantasy is by communicating. Fantasies are something that couples can enjoy together, to get each other aroused, and to have orgasms. You may not need a fantasy to get aroused but at some point while you're having sex you might want to experiment and incorporate some sexual fantasies.

Some people have to fantasise to have an orgasm but that doesn't mean the fantasy is removing you from your partner, you may tap in and out of your sexual fantasy depending on what your sexual exploration looks like at the time.

There are so many different ways of becoming aroused or turning each other on; the idea of teasing each other. We never take enough time with foreplay and it is often seen as a tedious step to get to the actual sexual act. Because sex happens in the brain it takes a while to forget about work, deadlines, or life in general, so spending time in that foreplay zone can be hugely beneficial. Foreplay adds texture to the experience of sex.

The senses of sight, taste, smell and touch all play such an important role in getting us aroused and turned on, hence the huge number of products available with various scents and flavours. The products used are usually made with material that feels sensual and good on the skin and adds a layer of excitement where people can stay longer in the fore-play zone.

No one is saying there is no place for quickies but the more you can master communicating during foreplay in terms of what feels good, how you want to be touched, and listening to how your body reacts or doesn't react, the more the experience of sex will be overall. Taking the time without the involvement of penetration or genitals helps with communication and listening to one another. A lot of the time people do say what they like and what they don't like but are they actually listening to what their partner likes?

Spending time in foreplay can help you both relax, ease anxieties, improve intimacy and affirm each other and is a time to explore the different ways of having sex. Discussing whether to use sex toys and if so, which ones and if you're going to be using condoms and when to put it on, these details can all form part of foreplay.

We have to feel confident enough to say what type of sex we want, regardless of where you are in the process. The earlier the better so that

194

you can, for example, go together to buy condoms if you need them or check that the condoms you have haven't expired, grab the candles and feathers, put on the playlist and get in the mood.

Waiting till the heat of the moment can be problematic and many people feel pressure to continue even though they may not want to, so foreplay is a good time to talk about these practical, but extremely important, issues such as consent, filming or taking pictures, expectations after sex, etc. This is often the time when people consent to different types of foreplay or kissing and so it is at this point you can tell your partner to stop something you are not enjoying or if they signal whether it feels good or not.

Foreplay can set the tone for what someone can look forward to once there is penetration. Often we don't feel like we can say when something feels awkward during foreplay, yet sex can start and end at any point and we should all accept when a partner says they need a time out and stop. In terms of consent, there is often a heavy burden placed on the person who does not want to carry on with sex, whether it is during foreplay or penetration, but respecting those boundaries are non-negotiable.

The body is an erogenous zone so nibbling on the ear or the neck, having the face, breasts, nipples, forearm, inner forearm, elbow, torso, chest, umbilical area, groin and inner thighs, back of the knee, or even the toes, kissed, sucked, licked or teased, turns people on.

Having a variety of sensual materials that one can use for the touch sensation could include a silk tie, soft linen, leather or rubber. The differences in material elicit a different tactile experience. Caressing someone with a silky scarf creates a complex heightened nerve sensation that is not quite a tickle whereas a soft feather can give someone the sensation of being teased. A feather can be tantalising to use when caressing the back of the body.

Black leather, together with latex lubricants, are some of the biggest elements of erotic imagery or fantasy objects. Some people really like the feel of leather on their skin, whether that be gloves, a corset, a skirt or other items, and find that feeling sensual.

The stimulation that comes from various materials causes the body to feel different sensations and where someone may like a feather being stroked across their back, they might respond very differently to candle wax being dripped on their nipple. Explore with different material on different parts of the body.

The tongue is key when experimenting with different feelings and sensations and because it is usually at core body temperature, the warm, moist texture while flicking it over the skin can be enticing and elicit goosebumps and sensual feelings across the body. Roll your tongue around the nipples, the ears, and in circling motions around the belly button and lower back. Doing the same with ice in your mouth can also be incredibly sensual and can provide a complete contrast in sensation.

There are different ways you can get your body to be sensorily awakened and another aspect people don't consciously think about, or remember, is how you breathe. Blowing warm air onto the skin, at the back of the neck or somewhere around the armpit area, inner thighs or groin area is all that some people may be comfortable with initially.

There is always room for more experience and exploration and the very simple art of using your fingers to feel your partner's body or facial features such as tracing your finger around the outer margins of their lip or brow area, can be the start of other areas of experimentation. Sometimes you might not be consciously engaging in the tactile stimulation you are giving the other person but it can help in your own pleasure to be aware of what you are doing, whether it be moving your fingers tenderly around your partner's breast area and seeing what is comfortable for your partner and how it may actually turn you on if you focus on it.

The only way you'll know is by doing it and by lingering a bit longer on the body to really get to know your person. Light strokes over the abdomen, the lower back, on the thigh, adds to the excitement and the tease. This may also be the perfect time to talk about the common theme of sexual fantasy of being spanked or tied up, or your eyes being covered with a cloth or a tie. Fantasies do not have to be exceptional and not every fantasy can, or has to, come true but they can add intimacy to a relationship. Spanking, bondage and being restrained introduces a level of vulnerability and trust one has to have in your partner.

It's important to have a discussion beforehand about dominant play and the submissive role and agree on what it would look like. These conversations need to happen regularly and the people involved have to *always* be in agreement. I often tell people not to feel bad if they don't know what they want when it comes to bondage and spanking, etc., as it is a great opportunity to find out with your partner what consent is around bondage and the rules around it. It offers you an opportunity to do something with your partner of finding out different ways of experimenting and exploring together.

Not everyone is a virgin when they start a new relationship and this doesn't matter because each person is different and so you 'meet' their pleasure mannerisms and certain ways of having sex as you get to know them. Not all people who have sex are couples or desire long-term relationships, however those who are coupling, learning how to please each other and learning the lines of respect and what sex will look like for the two of you, is an important foundation for a relationship.

Domination and bondage is all about role playing and offers amazing possibilities for foreplay, exploring each other and sex. Talk about what kind of behaviour or performance turns you on, what you want and do not want to happen, the depth, speed, etc. and then colour in the details and stick to those guidelines. You have to have a signal or code word that both of you can recognise as a sign to stop the fantasy play and you both need to respect that moment and those boundaries.

If you have a bed with a headboard, you can delicately tie your partner's arms to it in such a way that they can untie themselves if they want to. Learning to tie knots is important in terms of remembering where the blood vessels are in the body and what to do over the joints, abdomen and neck and knowing which knots to use for the different types of play. Restricting someone's movement can be liberating for them as they are forced to pay more attention to what is happening to their body

Knotting 101

It's time to put your Girl Guide/Boy Scout training to the test! (I bet you never thought those knot tutorials would come in handy for *this!* ☺)

Here are some basic knots to get you started.

For those that want to tie up loose ends ☺ the square or reef knot is a good choice for rope bondage as it applies less pressure to the skin. It is used to tie two ropes together or to tie both ends of the same rope.

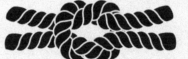

Reef knot

For those a bit more adventurous or experienced, a bowline knot is good for binding the wrists and ankles. It is a safe option as it can be loosened and will not cause nerve or blood supply constriction.

Bowline knot

and so it can be a fantasy for the dominant person as well as the person being restrained.

Some people fantasise about knee-high boots and perhaps a dominant might want to wear those boots as part of your fantasy. Your character can be informed by other sexual fantasies and exploring different 'characters' makes fantasy exciting.

The 'typical' master and slave roles can be reversed where the more dominant person in the day-to-day relationship can become the submissive one in the sexual fantasy play and vice versa. Dressing up, using a leather whip, incorporating vibrators and using lube can all be used to assert dominance and add to the thrill of the experience. Soft scarves and ropes can bring heightened arousal and can help in getting into playing the role of the dominant.

In discussing how these roles will play out, maybe the submissive person will beg for more or maybe the dominant person takes the lead and the partner goes with the flow. When it comes to the issue of submission, there is a certain level of obedience that is assumed, where, for example, the dominant gives instructions to kiss and caress and the submissive does so without complaint and with complete obedience.

Everything needs a form of discussion beforehand about respecting the rules of the game. If your mouth is not closed, communication is ongoing.

When it comes to what sexual play looks like there is no one way, no right or wrong, only what works for you. Communication is key, stick to the rules of the game and what you have agreed to, listen to each other, and most importantly, have fun! And remember, foreplay, foreplay, foreplay.

Communication during sex

Are you talking during sex? What are you saying? These are some of the first questions I ask during sex therapy and the answer will often tell me how confident that person is and gives me insight into the relationship dynamic. This applies to both individual and couples therapy. Often, people can feel disempowered, hurt, or neglected when they feel their opinion doesn't matter, or their needs are not being taken seriously even after expressing what they want.

It's human nature not to see the links between what happens in everyday life or the mundane and how those tensions or good habits affect libido, enjoyment and how people express or withhold intimacy, when people have sex and want to be intimate. The word 'intimate' has come to mean different things and I believe one can experience intimacy, bonding and profound joy even within casual relationships.

It's a fact that sex is not always attached to the need to maintain a relationship as a result of sex and not all sex is deep and meaningful; people have casual sex, they have friends with benefits, while others are sex workers, and intimacy means very different things in these scenarios and to these people.

Often, when relationships hit a rut, intimacy becomes a buzzword and it is said to be 'lacking'. Depending on what the issue is, this can be one of the first areas to show that indeed there is a break in the bonding and communication in the relationship.

And when I say talking, I'm not even referring to talking dirty (btw why do we call it 'talking dirty'? I think we need to find new words for it), I'm talking about the role of sound during sex. A lot of adults live in homes where there are children so they have to learn to have sex quietly. Sex is therefore literally 'silent' due to the actual spaces people are having sex in.

Spatial planning is so important; people having decent spaces to live in and how much of that is tied to dignity and to the fact that having sex is part of the healthy human experience, and how many adults are able to have sex in their own home without exposing children to inappropriate sexual content.

This is where sex sometimes becomes political, when we talk about human dignity and sex as a human right. When townships were being designed, it wasn't just a matter of racial injustice, there was so much more that was taken away from people. A home consisted of one room with a curtain that separated the kitchen from the main bedroom, so where did people have sex? In Johannesburg, so many people come to the city in search of gold but where are they all having sex in this overcrowded place? This is a basic, obvious observation but it boils down to the dignity given to each and every person.

At an AIDS conference held in Durban years ago, I was chair of the Department of Health's session that consisted of a panel of people from Johannesburg of different ages, genders, races, and sexual experimentation all talking about their sexual lives.

This made me think about the different types of sex people are having in Joburg, the different conditions attached to the type of sex and the actual places people are having sex. Johannesburg is still that city in Africa where a lot happens and a lot of people come to Joburg for business and business happens in many forms.

Linking this all to sex and sound, it made me think that of all these people having sex, who is allowed to express pleasure during sex? The issue of policing of women's sensuality and experimentation, sexual excitement, desire and fulfilment is a societal bias that is very much in force today. A lot of women I know are having sex silently, they are having orgasms in silence because they don't want to be seen as 'loose' or 'slutty' or having 'too much experience'.

A lot of sex still happens in the context that sex is being *done* to women and that dynamic often determines what sexual play tends to look and sound like. If we think back to our own experiences, for example while masturbating, it feels great to talk to yourself while masturbating. That is the space where you can become comfortable with your own voice and talking erotically and it can start with sounds of what feels good.

Moaning and groaning is a good way of giving feedback during sex so try it by yourself first and see if you enjoy it and whether it is something you wish to act out on someone else. You can have deep meaningful conversations during sex but moaning and groaning teaches someone that when you make certain sounds they mean something. You have to speak to each other and tell each other the sounds that made you feel good, ask what sounds made the other person feel good, so that you understand each other's sounds and almost come up with your own language during sex.

The so-called dirty talk is one of the ways that can enhance your sexual experience and the feedback lets your partner know that what they're doing feels good. It could be a whisper in the ear that perhaps turns into a nibble but by being vulnerable in that moment, it adds something deeper to the relationship.

There is nothing negative about people who talk during sex or who verbalise their fulfilment during sex. Pornography over-emphasises dirty talk so it can be seen as a turn-off for sex. If you are going to use pornography as your standard of what is to be expected during sex, you may find yourself underwhelmed and your sexual expectations might not be fulfilled.

Some people are introverted so it is unfair to expect them to talk dirty during sex when they may not talk much at all. For someone else, it may be part of their sexual fantasy to be more verbal during sex. At lot of women say they want to talk dirty but their male partners judge them for using dirty language. What is acceptable for one person might not be acceptable for another but the point is to give it a chance and try.

Talk to yourself when you masturbate, see how it sounds, how it makes you feel and then try incorporate it with your partner. Start off mild and work your way up to hardcore instruction of what you want. It can be something as simple as, 'I like your body/your lips', or 'Put your head between my thighs'. The only way to get used to talking dirty is to start talking! You may feel awkward and self-conscious, you might even giggle but keep going.

Use things to inspire you such as music, words, writing; there is no shortage of erotic material available. You might include poetry and erotic literature to your play, it just depends on different types of communication and comfort zones. Remember that what works for one partner doesn't always work for another. Talking dirty, coupled with tactile sensations, while giving or receiving feedback, can do wonders for your sexual experiences. It could even add to a sexual fantasy you didn't even know that you were interested in. Talking dirty and making sounds during sex is underrated and people don't realise how good it can be to hear what the other person wants; it makes the experience more fulfilling and rich.

Imagine having phone sex and while you aren't physically in the same location as your lover, phone sex can be romantic and it can be rewarding. It can improve bonding and intimacy and because of the level of trust required, it can make your sexual experience so much better. Remember though, people can record without your consent so make sure you have the conversation about getting the person's permission to record the conversation and the practicalities of what time to phone each other. Be as detailed in your descriptions as possible. Have foreplay during phone sex where you can masturbate or use video chat.

You might give your partner instructions during phone sex of what you would like them to do and that in itself can form part of fantasy or foreplay. Do this while your partner is at work before they come home. This build-up to the actual physical sex can be as important as the sex itself and the thrill of doing something naughty can be a huge turn-on.

If the trust is there you can put your mind to rest. If you are worried about your safety, about being recorded, or about your video landing up on the internet, this takes away from the pleasure in the moment. In that case, don't have phone sex and don't agree to be recorded. If you are feeling uncertain or uneasy, stop and make sure you only partake in phone sex or video calling when you feel safe and when you trust that the content doesn't land up in places you don't want it to.

Start simply, especially in the beginning. Use different tones and volumes and find out what excites your partner and what turns you on. Find those 'oohs' and 'aahs' and go for it. Don't think too much.

Overall, fantasy is private and it can remain private but there is space for couple exploration. The content shared should be inclusive of playful teasing and content that is fun for both partners. Together you can draw the picture, colour it in and share common fantasies. Playing games during foreplay, whether it be dice or adult cards, bondage, candle wax, giving each other massages, pretending you are a masseuse and your lover is overlooking a Caribbean beach, there is space for fantasy play to be done together and for the scenario to be built and for the details of it to be shared between the two of you.

When you have private fantasies don't feel guilty for leaving your partner in the dark. We shouldn't impose our own ideas of sexual imagery or fantasy onto someone else or try coerce our partners into acting the fantasies out if they don't want to. But fantasy can add a layer to your sexual lives. Send each other texts, voice notes, or emails during the day to build up the sexual tension. Play characters in the fantasy and make a location to 'meet'. Pause at a point in the fantasy and suggest surprises for when you meet up in real life. This all adds to the excitement and can add an exciting dimension to your sex life. So, go ahead, play!

What exactly is 'kink' and 'fetish'?

The world of kink is vast and not all that daunting and there are various ways you can slowly start exploring the world of kink. Beginner kink activities can slowly be incorporated into your sexual experimentation. Kink is considered to be more adventurous and is meant to enhance the experiences and sensations of the people taking part in sexual play. Kinksters can derive excitement from simple things incorporated into foreplay such as someone wearing stockings and lace or using candle wax, to the use of rope and gadgets involved in the spectrum of bondage, dominance or sadomasochism.

A fetish may involve a specific fantasy and a deep desire for objects or activities such as wearing nappies, and usually an obsession with non-genital body parts, such as toes or noses. Some fetishists may

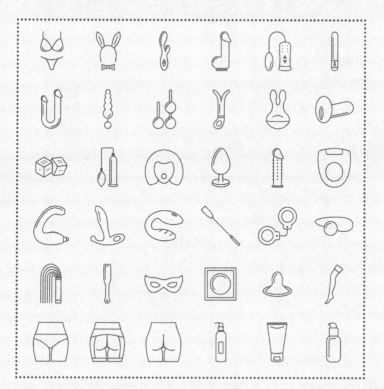

require a more detailed re-enactment of their fantasy in order to find sexual fulfilment and orgasm. Some fetishes may be on the edge of what is socially and legally unacceptable, especially when the content is enacted.

Blindfold

Using a material such as a tie, an eye shield or a scarf as a blindfold blocks out the light, thereby cutting off any visual stimuli. From foreplay to full-on sex, blindfolding makes it easier to focus and experience the touch sensation because you do not know what is going to happen next, or where, the anticipation can heighten the experience.

Hand ties

A range of materials, such as a scarf, a tie, or a loosely tied rope can be used for bondage. Aim for the ties to be tight enough around the wrists to restrict the range of motion but they must not hurt. Restricting the range of movement in the hands almost forces the person to go into the 'I can't do anything but enjoy the moment and receive pleasure' mode. Women often find they are able to tolerate this form of play well while receiving oral stimulation and when the roles are reversed, this can make them feel more dominant and in control.

Biting, scratching, candle wax and spanking

These sensations create a contrast to gentle touch and can result in shivers and a jolt of energy through the body. While at the height of arousal and the most turned on, the pain associated with these actions are experienced differently and the increased tolerance can result in an intense experience. The neck, the shoulders, the backs of the knees, and nipples are erogenous areas that respond well to gentle biting and scratching.

Aftercare is important when it comes to kink and describes the intentional process of checking in and debriefing after a kink session. It often involves discussing what worked for you as an individual and as a couple, what didn't work, the peak of enjoyment and reassuring each other what you would like to try again.

#TeamLayATowel

••

Sexual desire naturally fluctuates throughout a woman's menstrual cycle. For some, the changes in hormonal levels may result in premenstrual syndrome (PMS). The pelvic and lower abdominal pain caused by menstruation can be severe and management with pain medication can be most useful if taken before the pain reaches high levels.

During menstruation, as the lining of the uterus sheds, prostaglandins are released by the lining. These groups of compounds produced by the body have varying hormone-like effects, most notably the promotion of uterine contractions. Prostaglandins circulate in the blood and as part of their role, support the functions of platelets involved in blood clotting.

Prostaglandins also promote inflammation, pain and fever, which may explain the feeling of unwellness, especially in the early days of a period. On the first day of the menstrual period, the levels of the prostaglandins are high and as the days pass and the lining of the uterus continues to be shed, the levels decrease. As a result of the decrease, pain and other symptoms associated also usually decrease and one starts to feel better again.

This is the reason why much of the pain medication prescribed for period pain are the non-steroidal anti-inflammatory drugs (NSAIDs) because they specifically target prostaglandins. By acting on prostaglandins, they work by reducing the amount of prostaglandins in the bloodstream and therefore they reduce their effects. The effectiveness of NSAIDS make menstrual cramps less severe. The use of NSAIDS must be in consultation with a health provider because in prolonged use or high doses, they may cause side effects ranging from mild gastrointestinal upset like diarrhoea, allergic reaction and more serious adverse effects such as an increase in stomach and intestinal ulcers, and perforation of the stomach or intestines.

In some women, together with PMS, they also experience an increase in sexual desire and enjoy sexual penetration during their period. Yes, some women enjoy sex during menstruation. The interplay and resulting fluctuations of estradiol, progesterone and testosterone result in a hormonal orchestra and the desire for sexual activity and pleasure may last well into menstruation.

I am the self-proclaimed patron of #TeamLayATowel and I know the benefits first-hand. It may not always be that one feels ecstatic and eager to have sex but if you have had a positive experience with the post-orgasmic benefits of having period sex, one may be inclined to have it as one of the 'home remedies' for menstrual tension. The choice to have sexual penetration is a personal one; masturbation is also great. It may help allay some concerns regarding the amount of blood and the pain threshold involved in period sex. Many women notice a difference and the surge in their desire for sex at certain times in their cycle. The desire for intimacy and sex around ovulation is also known and a recognised part of a normal cycle.

It is possible to get pregnant during period sex because ovulation may happen soon after the period in those with shorter menstrual cycles, and the risk of STIs remain, therefore condoms should still be used. Remember sperm can survive up to seven days.

The benefits of having sex during a period is that having an orgasm may help relieve menstrual cramps. The tension in the pelvic area can be soothed and improved by a warm bath or shower before sex. Although there may be a slight increase in the flow immediately and soon after sex, it is short-lived and is not a problem. Some people may even have a shorter cycle due to the constriction of the blood vessels during sex.

I have spoken about #periodsex on Twitter and on the radio many, many times as I like to talk about it as a way to destigmatise menstruation. But also women's menstruating vaginas, as with many topics that are still taboo about sexual pleasure-related issues, especially sex during menstruation, is in the top five. Despite the world-wide religious and cultural restrictions placed on menstruating women, sex during a period is safe. Women are not dirty during menstruation nor is sex during a period sinful, weird or unhygienic. It is a personal choice.

Tips from the patron of #TeamLayATowel:

If you are a novice, start by having sex in the shower or bath

Lay a towel

Use darker sheets

Remove a cup or tampon before penetration

You may use a condom

You may require a lubricant. Water-based lubricant is safer especially for shower or bath sex as silicone may cause excessive slipperiness in water.

Anal play

Sex, sex, sex. A taboo topic but anal sex is probably one of the biggest topics that elicits uncomfortable responses and intrigue. A lot of people try to explore anal sex before reading up on it which can mean a lot of people's first attempts at anal play/sex is uncomfortable. It is then difficult to get someone to relax and enjoy it and thereby break some of the taboos surrounding anal play.

Because it is the anal area, a lot of people are concerned about germs, but with regular grooming, washing and cleaning, the area around the anus and perineum is no dirtier than any other part of your body. When people start to become inquisitive about anal sex, they ask how to prepare for it. More specifically, the receiver wants to know about cleanliness.

When talking about anal sex and preparation, the most important aspect is lubrication. The anal mucosa does not provide as much lubrication and moisture as, for example, those secreted in the vagina. Extra lubrication is recommended to enhance pleasurable and safer anal sex; without lubrication the risk of discomfort, pain and anal tears is greatly increased. Water-based lubricants remain a great option, are most accessible and should be used. They are also easier to clean up but they tend to get absorbed a lot quicker and if anal play lasts a long time, you may opt for a longer lasting silicone option. If you can get a silicon-based lubricant that is also effective to use with your choice of condoms, use it.

Getting ready for anal sex and how to clean the area ☺

A lot of people use anal douching; a liquid enema that cleans out the lower rectum and anal canal. The process takes a few minutes and the more you do it, the quicker and easier it gets. An enema is not always necessary if you have regular bowel movements as it means you are emptying your lower rectum. 'Over-using' douches and enemas can cause irritation and discomfort. It is best to read up on how to improve your diet, such as eating more salads, smoothies, fruit and vegetables for fibre, in the preparation leading up to anal play. If you are engaged in anal play on a regular basis, you might want to consider more specific dietary advice for longer term preparation in terms of lifestyle and a high fibre diet. To cleanse the area, take a few extra moments and use your finger while you are showering to clean out the lower end of the rectum.

A lot of people mistakenly think that anal sex is devoid of risk and because the risk of pregnancy does not exist, the use of condoms is not necessary. Many of the common STIs can be transmitted during anal sex, from oral play and penetration. HIV, specifically, has a higher risk of transmission through anal sex as opposed to vaginal sex. Making sure that the condoms you use are compatible with the lubricant you choose is vital.

If you are physically and emotionally tense about anal sex, the harder it will be to be relaxed enough for ease of penetration and this will also be evident in the tightness of the anal sphincter.

Visual learning is key, so get a mirror and use your finger to feel what the tension is around your anus, so that you know what it looks and feels like when someone else touches it. Practice breathing exercises with deep inhalations and exhalations prior to exploring anal play with a partner.

Solo anal play is encouraged before including partnered anal play. As you inhale, tense the muscles around the anus and when you exhale, relax the muscles. As you exhale and release the tension, take your finger and slide it into your anus, to see what it feels like. There shouldn't be pain, just a little pressure, as pain would mean that you are pushing too hard and too far.

It is best explained as graduated penetration and I always use the analogy of one centimetre per hour for beginners. Even when using a sex toy, a penis or any other object, you shouldn't advance insertion too hard, too deep or too fast. One centimetre per hour is usually the most comfortable option, as well as being the safest. If you are able to advance your finger with ease, sometimes quickly and deeply, because the girth of your finger is quite small, you will probably be able to advance your whole finger.

The differences in girth of the various objects used for insertion will change the experience and comfort level and staying comfortable and enjoying the sensation is important. The aim is not always to get full penetration the first time or even every time, but spending time in the comfort zone before you move from there is important for the overall experience.

The use of a finger as foreplay and the main play is encouraged and one can experiment by moving your finger in and out and around in circles as all of these movements change the pleasure. A lubricant is important even if you are exploring on your own and you may even want to wear a latex glove depending on your comfort level. Feel the inside of the anal canal and differentiate between the different types of tissue on the anal wall.

If you are a woman, and used to fingering yourself, you will feel easily the difference between the vaginal canal and the anal canal. Squeeze the sphincter on your finger to feel the sensation and that in itself can give a pleasurable feeling and you will also then know how to respond. The issue of being tense is the biggest factor when it comes to anal penetration or advancement and the tenseness of the anal sphincter can lead to an anti-climax and general loss of interest in sex.

Do not go beyond your comfort zone; the anal area is sensitive on both the outer and inner areas therefore do not push yourself, or your partner, beyond what is comfortable. There should be no straining or pain and the more relaxed, prepared and safe you feel, the better anal play exploration will be.

We often think sex is something that happens in the genital area only and in isolation, however your whole body is involved. The stages of early sexual arousal and excitement, with the accompanying vaginal lubrication, clitoral engorgement or the erection and maintenance of the erection, are all happening at the same time as well as other changes happening in the body such as the nipples becoming hard and engorged. People know they want to be touched in certain erogenous areas of their body because of this reaction to sensual stimuli.

The anal area and anal tissue is just as involved in the sexual excitement stage while having sex and during the climax while achieving an orgasm. As much as the vulva, the vaginal canal and the penis become rich and engorged with blood and ready for sexual play, the same response happens in the anal area. Aside from the need for lubrication, the anal area is just as responsive in sexual excitement and pleasure, as the rest of the pelvis. The nerve supply to the pelvis also supplies the anus and anal area.

Anal play can be as simple as using your lips or tongue to stimulate the anal area and anal sphincter. Some people insert the tip of their tongue into the anus and that can be quite pleasurable. Choosing to use a butt plug, anal beads or a small vibrator, all depends on your comfort level and what you become accustomed to.

For those with a prostate, the stimulation of the prostate gland can be done by gradually inserting a finger, a dildo, or a penis a few centimetres into the rectum. The stimulation in the anal area is different for women but equally enjoyable, even if they do not have an actual prostate gland to be stimulated. Some people specifically enjoy prostate orgasms and do not require any other type of sexual stimulation to achieve an orgasm.

The prostate area is usually known as the g-spot in males, whereas for women the area referred to as the g-spot is within the vaginal canal. The sensations that accompany a prostate orgasm can be felt in the same intensity as those of a g-spot orgasm. Whether anal play is happening to a man or a woman, women find anal sex just as pleasurable because the nerve supply, pelvic movements, lubricants, and the emotional and erotic experiences add up and play an important role in achieving an orgasm.

By stimulating the anal area externally and internally, in different positions and incorporating fantasies or toys, orgasms can be extraordinary and a lot of people have described them as unlike any other they've experienced. Some go as far as having anal play reserved as part of special moments such as birthdays, anniversaries and others enjoy it much more frequently. But it is also okay to not want to explore anal play at all.

Anal play, as with a lot of sexual pleasure, has nothing to do with a person's gender or sexual orientation and should be enjoyed by those who want to and on their terms. The more you engage in sexual play that is rewarding, the more experimental you will become, the more trusting and comfortable you will become.

Some couples engage in 'pegging' where a woman uses a strap-on dildo to penetrate her partner anally. The pegging of a man by a woman wearing a strap-on dildo is a fantasy for many heterosexual men. Sexual fantasy and sexual preferences should not be linked to gender identity or sexual identity. How a person finds sexual pleasure and gratification doesn't change who they are.

The sexual play of incorporating toys and being able to shop online in private means there is much more available for people to experiment with. Pegging is one of many examples of sexual play that can involve both partners and is a way to accept anal penetration as being normal for both parties and anal play, not always necessarily penetration, something to be normalised. If you are with a man who wants to have anal penetration and wants you to wear the strap-on and perform the penetration, it can take a bit of getting used to in terms of processing the request and taking on the role.

As such, the 'traditional' roles are reversed because often when we talk about anal play the assumption is that women are the ones receiving anal play and that all the preparation around anal tone and relaxation techniques is something to be mastered by women in hetero-sexual relationships, or men having sex with men or gay men. However, a lot of men enjoy anal play and the idea of getting penetrated by their lover, who is a woman, is a turn-on.

Nothing is for certain when having sex and the more open-minded people are, the more they can fantasise and bring their fantasies to life, in solo sexual pleasure or partnered with someone who is eager to explore.

Girl on girl

....

When it comes to sex between two women, people presume it is as easy as A-B-C or that it is incredibly difficult. Either way, sex is sex and women having sex with other women (WSW) is a valid form of sexual play. That there is no penis-vagina sex takes nothing away from the experience. Not all women who are WSW have to identify as lesbian or bisexual and for many women, their first sexual experience, if you widen the definition of sex, was with another women.

The internalised homophobia that demands a narrow spectrum for sexual expression and sexual play for men, in order to prove and maintain heterosexuality, makes sexual fluidity in women more accepted than fluidity in men assumed to be 'straight'. Sexual play such as prostate massage, anal play and anal penetration are seen as things only desired, performed and enjoyed by gay men, yet another example of why patriarchy is bad, even for men. This ingrains homophobia even further because heterosexual men, who enjoy anal play, are suspected or referred to derogatorily by various words, as 'gay'. The denial of sexual fluidity and the enjoyment of the erogenous zones limits the possibilities for pleasure, expression and fulfilment.

It is unfortunate that so much mainstream pornographic production of lesbian sexual contact is for the heterosexual male gaze and is often seen as foreplay. The main cast members are usually femme women (a lesbian whose appearance and behaviour are seen as traditionally feminine), again, presenting a stereotype that others are more masculine-presenting lesbians. The question of 'who is the man' in the relationship, that many WSW and lesbian women encounter, shows that sex is still only seen within strict gender and sexual expressions and that those boxes must mimic heterosexuality.

Even people skilled at web searches and on how to optimise search results, will find it difficult to find information specific to WSW. In fact, halfway through page one of a general WSW Google search, the results centre men and their pleasure in the discussions on WSW pleasure. In addition, there is also a lack of African lesbian and WSW erotic material and it is for this reason that I shamelessly plug the incredible curators at Hub of Loving Action in Africa (HOLAA!). With its humble beginnings as a blog, it is an online and physical space where women and gender non-conforming people of all sexualities learn and share through workshops, dialogues, archiving, digital conversations, knowledge production, partnerships and awareness building. Their latest safe sex and pleasure manual covers a host of topics and even contains a few erotica stories.

WSW sexual play is filled with heat and endless possibilities but just because it is two women having sex, the issue of safe sex cannot be overlooked. This is important for all sex, whether it be penetrative, strap-on, dildo, finger sex or non-penetrative sexual contact as any time bodily fluids and skin-to-skin genital contact happens, the risk of contracting an STI exists. STIs such as herpes, HPV, chlamydia, gonorrhoea, and syphilis can be transmitted through oral sex. Thus the use of a dental dam is so important.

You can make your own dental dam by cutting both ends off the external 'male condom' and using the square piece of latex to create a physical barrier during oral sex in the vulva and using a separate one for the anal area. Applying a water-based lubricant onto the vulva prior to using the dental dam or latex square, enhances pleasure by aiding in the slipperiness and ease of motion of the tongue. Condoms must also be used when vibrators, dildos and strap-ons are used. If possible, each person should have their own vaginal and anal toys that are not shared.

It is not uncommon to wonder if you or your partner are doing the 'right' things, so remember, when you fantasise, share your desires and what feels good to you, thereby making it easier to please each other. Verbal and non-verbal cues are important indicators as to what your partner likes or doesn't like.

Not every woman who is WSW has a desire to experience penetration. For those who want to enjoy penetration, it is best to start by experimenting with a finger or two and then plan further exploration using a dildo or strap-on. A strap-on may require some practice, depending how well one can master the strokes and get comfortable wearing it. The many varieties available means that you need to purchase a toy that fits the comfort level of the person wearing it as well as the pleasure needs of the person receiving penetration. Adjustable harnesses for strap-ons are also available so it is probably best to start with a purchase accommodating of different sizes and shapes.

There are so many possibilities and so many ways of having great sex. The maximal point of enjoyment and fulfilment is possible when you are liberated in your mind, body and soul.

Section 3

Sexual Rights

Advocating for sexual rights

··

In 2017, I received an invitation to be on the Global Advisory Board for Sexual Health and Wellbeing (GABSHW). It came from the secretariat after they had done research to find out who in the region was doing work aligned to their vision and mission. The GABSHW is a body that was convened to do various thematic work on sexual health, sexual rights and sexual pleasure. To quote the GAB, 'the board aims to highlight the importance of considering sexual health, sexual rights and sexual pleasure equally and to provide a call to action to global organisations, policy makers, NGOs and governments to achieve a rights-based perspective on sexuality in policy, law, practice and research'. I was quite surprised as I didn't know there even was an advisory board such as this, but it was a welcome confirmation of how important the work is. At the time, it was one of the most exciting experiences for me because it was at a point in my career as a medic focusing on sexual health, when I was looking for my 'tribe'. I was doing content production and media work trying to destigmatise sex, sexuality, gender and sexual liberation for women. Sexual health is often discussed and happens through heterosexuality, but it happens on a hierarchy of a scale that puts male pleasure above all other pleasure.

When I was chosen to be a member of the board, I joined a team of board members from all over the world trained in research, law and clinical practice and medicine; I was part of the sexual pleasure revolution! Here I was in Johannesburg, carving out a path as a general practitioner with an interest in reproductive and sexual health, when the opportunity came up and I knew it was something that I couldn't turn down.

The first board meeting I attended was in London and it became clear to me right away that I was in good company. The advisory board was established in 2016 with a specific mandate; advocating for a more positive and inclusive approach of how we view sexuality. Sexuality is a basic part of the human experience and sexual rights play a big part in human rights. We can't divorce sexual pleasure and expression from the discussion on sexual rights because the principles and rights that affirm people's respect and dignity, self-worth and safety, are principles and rights of every aspect of our lives. If you can get it right in terms of sexual rights and wellbeing, you will get to a place where people can express themselves and enjoy their health and sexuality. The literal access to health service is important because the constitution protects these rights.

We need to be deliberate about continuous review of policy and translating policies into services that affirm people who interact with health services. This extends to promotion, prevention, and overall wellness that we can bring to the population.

Sexuality is complex, but not necessarily difficult. It encompasses so much of the personal but is also influenced by other external factors such as spirituality, cultural constructs, or moral concerns. When people hear the word 'sexuality', they are immediately on the defence as if it implies sexual acts or intercourse. Sexuality encompasses personality, social roles, gender and sexual identity and the expression of your gender. It is about thoughts and feelings and how we are able to cognitively process and understand our own sexuality in its fullness and completeness and understand it as such, even before we are sexually active with other people.

There are so many toxic and negative behaviours about sex and sexuality and that is the reason why my work over the last two years has been so deliberate, and why being part of the global advisory board has been fundamental to me talking about these behaviours and taking the steps to help change them. I've found myself in a space where the more visible I am and the more I speak and take part in these discussions, the more questions are directed at me.

In my reading, I found that some of the definitions around sex and sexual health were old, only around heterosexuality and about a man 'doing' something to a woman. And not nearly enough around sexual pleasure. I have always been fascinated about how we can have those conversations about sexuality and sexual health.

Huge amounts of money are spent on HIV campaigns annually, yet sexual pleasure is something that never ever features. It is always so frustrating for me to see how sexual pleasure disappears (or is often completely missing) from literature, public health campaigns, policy and public health plans and how medicalised sex and sexual pleasure is.

At The Global Advisory Board we created a working definition of sexual pleasure, with a specific bias, and we are quite proud of elevating sexual pleasure as a lens that we use to talk about sexuality. The definition, adopted in 2016, reads:

> Sexual pleasure is the physical and/or psychological satisfaction and enjoyment derived from solitary or shared erotic experiences, including thoughts, dreams, and autoeroticism. Self determination, consent, safety, privacy, confidence; the ability to communicate and negotiate sexual relations are key enabling factors to sexual health and well-being. Sexual pleasure should be exercised – particularly the right to equality, non-discrimination, and the right to the highest attainable standard of health. The experiences of human sexual pleasure are diverse and sexual rights ensure that pleasure is a positive experience for all concerned and not obtained by violating other people's rights.

We also adopt the WHO definition of sexuality and sexual rights because we all come from different parts of the globe, so it is important to have a common thread that binds us and that the rest of the world can recognise.

The WHO states:

The fulfilment of sexual health is tied to the extent to which human rights are respected, protected and fulfilled. Sexual rights embrace certain human rights that are already recognized in international and regional human rights documents and other consensus documents and in national laws.

Rights critical to the realization of sexual health include:
- the rights to equality and non-discrimination
- the right to be free from torture or to cruel, inhumane or degrading treatment or punishment
- the right to privacy
- the rights to the highest attainable standard of health (including sexual health) and social security
- the right to marry and to found a family and enter into marriage with the free and full consent of the intending spouses, and to equality in and at the dissolution of marriage
- the right to decide the number and spacing of one's children
- the rights to information, as well as education
- the rights to freedom of opinion and expression, and
- the right to an effective remedy for violations of fundamental rights.

The responsible exercise of human rights requires that all persons respect the rights of others.

The application of existing human rights to sexuality and sexual health constitute sexual rights. Sexual rights protect all people's rights to fulfil and express their sexuality and enjoy sexual health, with due regard for the rights of others and within a framework of protection against discrimination.' (WHO, 2006a, updated 2010)*

Our hope, as the GAB, is that sexual pleasure can retake its rightful place when discussing sexual rights and sexual health, and that this pleasure revolution can complete the triangle in how we all approach sexuality; whether we are in research, policy or programmes.

I specifically themed this book into the three sections of health, pleasure and rights because of this and that as a first book, it is important to set the context and scene of the times that we are in, but also as a vision of what the future can look like. Looking at what is and where we are failing is important, but at the same time we need to have a vision of what the best is that we think we deserve.

We cannot talk about health and young people and sexuality and sex, and continue to neglect the issue of sexual pleasure. Auto-eroticism, commonly understood as masturbation, needs to be normalised as something that is not weird or bizarre but something commonly accepted. Sexual rights can be a positive bridge to bring us together and understand, as opposed to deliberately misinterpreting sexual rights to be people having a right to do whatever they want to other people.

Auto-eroticism is being sexually stimulated; arousal through stimulation of oneself or one's body and there are different ways auto-eroticism can take place. I am a big advocate for masturbation because if you do not know what feels good to you, how will you be able to tell someone else what you enjoy. Some people don't enjoy sex because of this exact fear and of being unsure how they will react, what will their body do. That anxiety of anticipation can work against you so when we talk about sexual pleasure, masturbation or auto-eroticism, it forms a big component of what that is.

Aside from the pleasure and rights issues, the principle issue talks about the approach to sexuality; the diversity. Diversity not just in our bodies but in life circumstances. It speaks to the issue of gender equality. Affirming sexual experiences for boys are not necessarily the same for girls who often don't enjoy the same normalisation of sexual experiences. The principles of sexual rights and sexuality speaks to autonomy and why it is important for people to have the information required to make decisions that can be life-changing.

It is so important, especially in the context of South Africa where so many people experience some form of harassment or trauma or rape, that we talk about the fact that sexual rights speak to the issues of violence, exploitation and abuse.

As much as we are advocating for sexual pleasure, for some people the journey of attaining the highest possible level of pleasure does involve some form of trauma. Do we have systems and emergent care for people who have gone through such forms of abuse? Not accepting that sexual pleasure is a right that every individual has, might explain why we don't provide services to victims of sexual abuse or violence. Services that are non-judgemental and affirming and where the content of programmes are respectful and take into account different cultures and religions and where personal beliefs are not forced onto the people asking for expert help and advice. We need to listen and be more attentive to what clients need and the issue of confidentiality is tantamount.

Very often in the rural communities and local clinics there are questionnaires asking if young people are in need of youth services and the overwhelming response would be that it is but there is the element of trust involved in that. Going to a clinic labelled 'youth friendly' would mean that perhaps your information will be used in some way and not kept confidential. We often don't think enough about what makes us decide to go to a certain doctor and not another.

I have patients who tell me they have a family doctor but if it involves their sex life they would rather come to me. This makes me wonder what is it about our different needs that makes people refrain from seeking assistance or seeking assistance from someone in particular?

People have a right to choose who they want to confide in and it doesn't matter where you go in the world, there should be services that take into account your lived experiences and that can be provided in a dignified manner, so that we know the quality people receive is of a high standard.

This brings to me to the question of where are young people getting their information on all of these concepts? Structured and comprehensive sexual education is desperately needed that will provide young people with an understanding of sexuality and emotional psychosocial factors. Often when we don't understand something, we tend to get defensive.

Parents who are not recipients of affirming approaches to sexuality often question what information their children are given in school. This brings an interesting element to how do we redress the gaps that we as parents or caregivers have that result in us not being able to transfer the knowledge in a positive manner?

We cannot talk about sex without talking about respect. Respect and consideration for people, how they enjoy sex and how they want to experience pleasure. We operate in a society that has very strong ideas about culture and religion, where a lot of people live very scripted sexual lives to fit into a box and do not learn about their body or what feels good. When you don't know how to listen to yourself or take a moment to re-energise yourself, how can you make your partner feel good?

When people get it right in terms of sexuality and sexual expression, all of the benefits spill over into other areas of our lives. For many people when things go wrong, rights are violated related to their sexuality, reproductive and sexual health, some of those consequences are lifelong. How is it that as a society we still continue to underplay the importance of sexual rights, sexual health and sexual pleasure, knowing they are intertwined and that the triangle needs to be in balance?

Depoliticising sexual rights has to be resisted precisely because all aspects of our lives, particularly sexual and reproductive health and the obsession with the fertility of women is political.

Many years ago, I started watching video lectures and clips of both Professors Kimberlé Crenshaw and Loretta Ross, as they delivered various talks, lectures and commencement speeches. Both professors are African-American women and their work, lived experiences and scholarship have moved me deeply and influenced and shaped my work the most.

Through their work, I started to engage with the principles of

Reproductive Justice and Intersectionality. In June 1994, twelve women of colour, Professor Loretta Ross being one of them, working in the reproductive health and rights movement, birthed the concept of reproductive justice at a pro-choice conference on healthcare reform in Chicago. Drawing on black feminist and critical legal theory from 1989, Professor Kimberlé Crenshaw developed the legal framework of intersectionality, a term that speaks to the multiple social forces, social identities, and ideological instruments through which power and disadvantage are expressed and legitimised.

All these years later, I find myself as a black woman in South Africa, finding sisterhood via the interweb with the women of colour in the United States, learning from their scholarship. I didn't foresee how deeply rooted my work as a medical doctor would turn into advocacy and even on a clinical level, I could feel the gaps regarding where to locate my work and once I understood what Reproductive Justice was, I saw immediately how intersectionality was the bridge to justice.

The universe conspired and I have since met both Professors Crenshaw and Ross and had the privilege of spending time with them and the way they received me, affirmed me and my work, was testament to the healing power of black love.

More than the birds and the bees

As strange as it may sound, I never thought I would be 'Dr T the Sex Doctor'. As much as it seems very intertwined and natural, I didn't always have a clear picture in my mind, but there is something to be said about surrendering to what you believe in. The whole 'what should I drag, what should I drop' concept.

That moment for me really crystallised during my community service year in 2010. The first point of clarity that I had about what kind of legacy I would want for myself as a medical doctor fell into place, but at the time I hadn't made the connection between the self and passion and how your passion can be work and can feel like you are doing something meaningful every day.

While working in community clinics on the West Rand of Johannesburg, I started by performing typical primary healthcare consultations. It soon became very clear to me that something was happening in the consultation rooms that nobody was aware of. I started to notice that patients, who seemed to understand their chronic disorders such as diabetes or epilepsy, or sexually transmitted infections, would leave the consultation seemingly clear and 'buy' into their treatment plan but would return days, weeks or months later with a worsening of their disease, or having not followed through with certain aspects of lifestyle changes.

This showed there was a breakdown somewhere along the line. I felt confident that as a doctor I had explained everything to my patients and covering all areas of concern, but in light of the trend I became more deliberate in asking questions about challenges they faced, after the consultation, the longer the consultations became. I had to spend more time finding out from the patients what the elements were that were informing their decisions, when it came to their health. Because I presumed they understood what was expected of them in terms of their care, I couldn't understand why they were still making what the medical field calls 'bad' decisions regarding their health.

When it came to the sexual health side of things, it soon became apparent to me that it was the area health workers were letting patients down on the most. For example, many of the questions posed to patients during a sexual history is about the number of people a person is having sex with and there is almost always judgement from the healthcare worker based on that person's response. In that moment, patients feel exposed and judged and without even thinking consciously about it, decide whether a nurse or a doctor can be trusted and whether or not they are in a safe space. This impacts whether patients feel they can open up and be honest.

I started to think about asking patients what type of sex they were having, i.e. were they having anal sex, was there penetration involved, and if so, was there a toy or penis involved, are they engaged in oral sex only, and I stopped assuming the kind of relationships they were in. I thought about the different ways of speaking to someone, what kind of questions you needed to ask and therefore the quality of the answers you would receive.

I tested this on my patients, not asking them how many people they were sleeping with or if they were using a condom, but rather what makes sex feel good for them. By asking this, they had to stop and think about what role they took in sexual interactions with their partner(s). The next question I asked was often met with a lot of reservation, followed by a sunken look, especially by women, and a certain level of vulnerability that I wasn't always expecting and always caught me off guard.

The question was, 'Do you have sex when you want to have sex, and when you have sex, do you have sex the way you want to have sex?' This question revealed how many people had never actually thought that between sex starting and ending, did what happened in between actually feel good?

I found myself reading more about the psychology of sex and the issue of coercion came up over and over again. The issue of whose sex is this? Whose orgasm is this? The view was that sex was something 'done' to women was sustained through pop culture, music lyrics, movies and in general conversations. Sex is seen as something done to people who are seen to be less dominant or less powerful in a relationship and those people 'give it up'.

Feeding into this same idea, I always use the analogy to further explain how sex has become so devoid of all players. For many people 'sex starts with an erection and ends with an ejaculation', and that's all there is to it. Not only do we not communicate about what feels good in the moment, we also fail to negotiate foreplay and what happens after sex. People can feel an emotional anti-climax after sex if they want to cuddle but their sex partner is not interested, while some may be having a one-night stand and leave straight away.

There is so much involved around the details of what actually happens when we are having sex. The discussion on safer sex tools such as dental dams, condoms and contraception is vital. Not only are the numbers for STIs high in South Africa, but we are in the lead when it comes to new HIV infections and, in addition, we have a huge problem with antibiotic resistance bacterial STIs.

Safe sex tools and what is available in public spaces are geared towards people who have penises, i.e. men, but the burden of safe sex falls on people, i.e. women, who are not the ones who need to use the external condom (which used to be called the male condom). There are now five external 'male' condoms available in public places, where most people access condoms. The public health system has invested in procuring four scented condoms plus the older non-scented one.

For women, and those who may need to use the internal condom for anal sex, the design of the external condom has not been improved for comfort for many years and access to lubricant isn't that easy. How do we then have the conversation about safer sex when we still burden women with ensuring the proper use of male condoms, their availability and the negotiation of its use in the first place?

Because of 'stealthing', the rampant, unlawful and deceitful removal of a condom during sex, this places women at a disadvantage right from the start. The structural issues around the language used when talking about women needing empowerment, needs to be adjusted. Women do not need more empowerment to be able to have safer sex, they need access to their own safer sex tools that they can choose to use on themselves and understand the pleasure benefit thereof.

When an external condom is used incorrectly, it can result in pregnancy and so pregnant women bear the evidence of unprotected sex and stigma that follows the person's circumstances and what they then choose. We have to have the discussion as to how much promotion of sexual health and wellness are health systems committed to if the majority of people who are having sex do not have access to safer sex tools and our country continues to lead the world in HIV complications?

How much of those failures do we understand to be a violation of people's human rights? Sexual rights, sexual pleasure, sexual health and sexual wellbeing are all human rights. At what point does the system take responsibility for that as opposed to burdening the people who are most likely at risk of coerced sexual contact, those with less power to negotiate sexual contact, into ensuring that they practice safe sex?

One day a group of young women came into the clinic asking for internal condoms; back then they were still referred to as 'female condoms'. (In 2018, the FDA approved the renaming of the 'female condom' to 'the internal condom'.) The young women giggled and were embarrassed about it; behaviour to be expected from teenagers, and they were dismissed quickly.

I often think back to that event in that it was a missed opportunity for the healthcare provider to provide answers or advice or ask open-ended questions that could have led the young women to feel more at ease and find out more information. The women probably felt ignored and put off ever wanting to visit the clinic again. So many young people, the world over, continue to be denied information and services even when they reach out.

It can be difficult in some relationships to negotiate safer sex and as a society we are failing to assist young people, and by default ourselves, in the way safer sex discussions are framed because it is often framed that if you don't want to have sex now, or if you don't want to have sex without a condom, a relationship must end. Or that no is a sign of someone having to pursue or push harder. We need to respect self-determination and that if someone doesn't want to have sex in that moment, it does not mean that relationship is valued any more or any less and it is not a catastrophe.

Maybe in a few hours' time that person will want to have sex and at that time they should be in a space where they know their request can be fulfilled, if their partner also wants to have sex. There is a very important layer we miss when we discuss consent and relationships. A lot of young people feel they don't want to say no to their partner's requests for sex for fear of them breaking up with them.

We need to understand that masturbation and self-play are regarded as 'sex'. If someone has an erection, feels aroused and wants to be sexual, then masturbate or not, but an erection is not a permanent state and in fact happens spontaneously sometimes. Not every erection is a signal for sex. People need to know that they can have an erection and that the erection doesn't need an outlet that is another individual.

In a column I wrote for *Teen Vogue*, I spoke about my framing of sexual pleasure as a human right and my deliberate reasoning thereof. A lot of negative sexual experiences stem from the very basic idea of what consent is and isn't but it's also about respecting the people involved and the importance of the ability to self-determine. It is simple: there is no pleasure without consent or clarity or open and honest communication. There is no pleasure without a safe space where the person knows that should they not want to continue they will be respected.

We don't often think of sexual pleasure as a human right because, unfortunately, a lot of people equate sex with violence. Think about the word 'sex'. Sex is, by default, consensual. Anything that isn't consensual, isn't sex, and there are words for that, which is why language is so important as it gives meaning and to meaning we attach feelings and associations.

When one talks about sex and sexual pleasure it is about consensual sexual contact between people who within their own contexts, legally, are able to consent to sex. Anything other than that is coercive and is rape and we need to stop using references to 'sex' when describing rape.

In medical school unless you had a personal interest in sexuality and gender, and did your own extracurricular reading, the curriculum didn't equip me to speak to my peers, never mind patients seeking treatment. Without being able to turn to a health professional, young people turn to pop culture for guidance and information. For heterosexuals this may seem to help but for any other person with a different identity, this can be a dead end. There is so much in pop culture and media that neglects to highlight the importance of consent and safer sex and there isn't enough information in the mainstream to normalise healthy sexual behaviour and debunk myths.

I decided to use social media as an advocacy tool to provide sex positive health information. Research shows that the consequences of a lack of sex education is disastrous. This is throughout all age groups and manifests in different ways; the extreme lengths women are going to to 'clean' their vaginas in an effort to make it tighter or smaller, through to a patient diagnosed with hypertension who has noticed a change in their erection.

If you don't know that sexual pleasure is your right, how will you know how to talk about it as such? If you have been diagnosed with depression or have started using contraceptives and can see a change in your libido and sexual response, if you are dismissed when voicing your concerns to your healthcare provider, this can be discouraging and is often why people default on their treatment because sex feels good.

As healthcare providers we cannot dictate to people where to place sex for themselves in terms of its importance in their lives. Healthcare professionals may feel that controlling high blood pressure, for example, is more important than sexual pleasure but for a patient who isn't affirmed and enabled to have these discussions around pleasure and other options of treatment, at that moment sexual pleasure might be a more pressing issue for them. A person might feel that since starting certain medications, their erection is negatively impacted or clitoral stimulation is less and that is what is important to them. We know high blood pressure is often called a 'silent disease' so it is more difficult for someone to ignore a very real issue with their sexual pleasure and put their trust in the medication they may still not be convinced they need.

We can't talk about sexual pleasure without talking about the expectations of what it is to be sexual and how women are shamed for having sex, initiating sex, and, God forbid, enjoying sex. Sex happens within the hierarchy that places male pleasure very high. There is a negative undertone to what it means to be the type of woman who is sexually liberated and how promiscuity is imposed and presumed because a woman may be sex positive and body positive and is not shy to talk about self-play, masturbation or sex toys.

We must normalise and discuss self-play and masturbation as a way to explore our own bodies; where women can partake in genital massage and affirmative self-play without penetrative sex. Adults exceptionalise penetrative sex over other types of intimacy, such as kissing or dry humping, that can both lead to sexual stimulation and intimacy without penetration.

If we are only ever going to talk about sex as being penetrative and exclude women having sex with women and women penetrating men with sex toys, we will never explore the other ways of being sexual if we deny that there is more than one way of having sex or experiencing sexual contact. We need to work on and continue the sexual pleasure revolution in creating a world where sexual pleasure can find its rightful place in literature, medical care, lyrics and media production. Where we can give people the information required and normalise sexual behaviour. We need to depict what it is to give affirmative consent and have healthcare services geared towards liberating young people, not just young people but for everyone, wherever you may be on the rainbow, to define what good sex is.

Pop culture is so profound in its relevance to the era we are in and the world that I want to live in. The TV series, *Pose*, premiered in June 2018 and is an American dance musical set in 1980s New York City. It explores different layers and complexities of life and society in New York and the LGBTQIA+ youth take you through the journey of being rejected by their birth families and going to New York to make a life for themselves. Living in a house with a house mother and being the 'children' of the house, points to the idea of them taking care of each other at different stages of their journey of coming out and dealing with their sexuality.

There was a subculture of the LGBTQIA+ community in New York at the time, where the African American and Latinx ball culture was developing and each house member would judge each other based on their outfits, dance skills and drag categories. From all walks of life, the characters depict real human experiences and I found myself affirmed by the series in more ways than it just being pure entertainment.

In terms of my own personal journey, you don't watch *Pose* and come out unchanged. It is an invitation into people's lives and stories done in a respectful manner and is everything I think TV and drama should, and can, be about. It is incredible in showing how pop culture can be so important in affirming people and experiences, and being deliberate and unapologetic about centring people and those whose voices continue to be marginalised because of their gender, age and class.

The way society organises itself is the same way it is organised in the queer community and it highlights what all the roles mean in a world that is not heteronormative and can reference a wider experience of human sexuality. There is nothing more affirming than having transgender people play themselves. If you are a young person, adult, caregiver, parent, or are wondering where you fit in, *Pose* shows that you are not alone, you can be seen and heard, even about thoughts, fears and anxieties you didn't know you had.

When I run workshops and do training with undergrad doctors and nurses, *Pose* is a reference point I use about who we are as people and who the people are that we serve. It gives a better understanding of the different complexities some people need to suffer through just to breathe. *Pose* gives you a chance to feel seen. When you can find references that are affirming and don't caricature the queer community, I think it is so important to draw on these resources.

Resources can be in the form of a teacher, a doctor, a nurse, a faith-based leader or priest, a counsellor, but whoever that may be, it is my wish that everyone has someone to offer them that space to breathe and heal. To hear them, see them and affirm them. As we talk about sexual rights, sexual health and well-being and sexual pleasure, *Pose* should be mainstream and the new normal and truly encompasses what I am about and the world I envision.

Sex Education is a British comedy that premiered in 2019 and introduces us to a sexually awkward teenager called Otis. He is navigating the issue of relationships, while living with his mother who is a sex therapist. The dynamic adds a comedic layer to what would normally be a dull encounter with sex and sexuality between mother and child. Because Otis grew up around conversations about sex, it made him kind of an expert in the field and the series takes us through a lot of different experiences such as how to have your first sexual encounter.

LGBTQIA+ is a theme in the series which proves we can have programming and television with references to pop culture that are not hyper-sexualising, or problematising young people's inquisitiveness. Otis's friend, Eric, is a young man struggling with the issue of being gay and masculine, but who presents very differently in terms of clothing and how his parents, particularly his father, see him in terms of the fears around raising a child different to their gender expression. *Sex Education* handles issues with so much delicacy and thoughtfulness and is a great conversation starter for parents and caregivers. It depicts the reality we are living in and my wish is that such productions could be made available to everyone. Pop culture can absolutely capture, in a nutshell, the kind of world that we all deserve and should commit to as a reality.

I will assert again that sexual pleasure is a human right and by virtue of sex and pleasure it demands sexual contact, expression, desires and fantasies that are free from judgement, coercion, stigma and violence.

Sex work is work

··

I attended the United Nations General Assembly side events in September 2018 and, as has become somewhat of a tradition, I stayed on in Manhattan for a few days after the official programme to take in some of the magic that is New York City. I was walking across the street on Broadway and saw a massive billboard with *Pretty Woman* in neon red lights. I immediately felt nostalgic as *Pretty Woman* is one of my top two movies of all time. It was only a few weeks prior that I had watched the movie, for what must be the hundredth time, and had live Tweeted using the hook, 'sex work is work' as I indulged in the movie.

For anyone who hasn't seen the movie (which is highly unlikely), the film centres around Vivian Ward, infamously played by Julia Roberts, and Edward Lewis, played by Richard Gere. Their first encounter sets the scene for a business transaction; the exchange is cheeky and happens on the street before Vivian agrees to leave with Edward. They navigate various issues during their week-long rendezvous and go on to develop a romantic relationship.

It was only when I had watched *Pretty Woman* a few times that I realised what the first encounter between them was really about; a businessman acquiring the services of an escort.

Although many people do not necessarily identify themselves as sex workers, sex work in its many forms is considered work. The adoption of the use of the term 'sex work' was in the 1970s and the International Labor Organization (ILO), a specialised agency of the United Nations, affirmed and recognised sex work as work.

In my work as a medical doctor and in the area of medical policy, many people in public health view sex workers through a narrow lens of HIV. This conjures gross stereotypes about sex work and sex workers as sex workers, in all the various gender and sexualities, are not 'vectors of disease'. Not all sex workers engage in sexual contact and those who do are not all performing penetrative sexual acts. Though, undeniably, that is a big part of sex work.

Not all sex workers are HIV positive and HIV is not the only concern that sex workers have. Public health does not need to be safeguarded from sex workers and even governments who boast HIV programmes for key populations at risk of HIV, still fail to provide lubricants and internal and external condoms and facilities remain inaccessible for the majority of sex workers. Sex workers have needs beyond HIV such as treatment of other sexually transmitted diseases, cervical cancer screening, trauma counselling, contraceptives and safe abortion care.

Sex workers face higher risks of HIV acquisition due to the criminalisation of sex work, sex workers and the clients. These continued hostile legal frameworks are a form of violence by states and contributes to the high level of stigma and discrimination. The discrimination is wide and inclusive of barriers to accessing financial and banking systems, safe working spaces, stigma in society and recourse and access to legal practitioners when rights are abused.

The need for states to protect, uphold and defend the rights of sex workers is an urgent global feminist issue. One that has been eclipsed by global health politics, economic crises and migration, yet these very issues are well documented as structural drivers of HIV, human rights abuses and women are always adversely affected. Global efforts have been growing in specific countries such as South Africa, led by the biggest sex worker-led movement, Sisonke, and the advocacy and policy work of SWEAT (Sex Workers Education & Advocacy Taskforce).

Dudu Dhlamini, a world-renowned activist living in Cape Town, is one of my mentors who has taught me so much about sex work, decriminalisation and feminism. In July 2018 at the International AIDS Conference in Amsterdam, I joined Dudu and many of our colleagues for what felt like yet another international talk-shop on the neglected cousin, sex work decriminalisation. Despite the cynicism, excitement was building for our celebration of Dudu as she was due to receive an award for her work as founder of the Mothers for the Future programme. The programme works hard to make sure sexual reproductive health is realised for sex workers and we were honoured to be there to celebrate with Dudu.

It was with much vigour that Sisonke, SWEAT and members of the Asijiki Coalition, were involved in a march in solidarity with PROUD, the Dutch union of sex workers in Amsterdam, as they delivered a memorandum to city officials demanding protection of the right of sex workers to work in safe working conditions in the city. We have been a part of several protests, highlighting several issues affecting women, and of course sex work decriminalisation, and at previous protests we resorted to throwing sanitary towels on stage to protest the VAT placed on sanitary products.

We cannot divorce the human rights of dignity, safety and bodily integrity from sex work. Sex worker rights are women's rights, health rights and labour rights and are the litmus test for intersectional feminism. The impact of continued criminalisation of the majority of sex workers, who are mostly women and transgender women, means that sex worker rights are a feminist issue.

We must all support the global demand for sex work decriminalisation and fund evidence- and rights-based intersectional programmes aimed at sex workers and their clients. Global and local feminists and organisations must support efforts to address structural barriers and ensure implementation of a comprehensive health service package for sex workers as advised by the WHO and fund public campaigns to decrease stigma.

In an op-ed recently published in *Teen Vogue*, I asserted that governments ignore the nuanced histories and contexts in different countries and thus continue to wrongfully offer blanket solutions and 'rescue' models which are rooting for partial decriminalisation or continued criminalisation of sex work. They also ignore the wishes of sex workers, who want full decriminalisation, as supported by the Global Commission on HIV and the law, and *The Lancet* journal, as well as human rights organisations like Amnesty International. They often fail to accept the evidence for the economic and social bases for sex work; the ILO estimates that 'sex workers support between five and eight other people with their earnings. Sex workers also contribute to the economy'.

As a medical doctor, I exchange payment in the form of money to provide people with advice and treatment for sex-related problems; therapy for sexual performance, counselling and therapy for relationship problems and treatment of sexually transmitted diseases. Basically, I am a sex worker.

I make this statement not devoid of the appreciation of the violent workplaces, or the harsh environmental conditions that outdoor sex workers endure and because of this privilege, I ask the question, is a medical degree really the right measure of who is deserving of dignity, autonomy, safety in the work place, fair trade and freedom of employment? No. This should not be so. Those who engage in sex work deserve those things too.

I do not believe it is right or just that people who exchange sexual services for money are criminalised and that I am not for what I do. Sex worker services can include everything from companionship, intimacy, counsel, to non-sexual role playing, dancing, escorting and stripping. It does not, I repeat, it does not always include penetrative sex. Many do not necessarily identify as sex workers, and that is also okay. Many take on multiple roles with their clients and some may get more physical while others may have started off as sexual may evolve into more emotional and psychological bonding. The clients vary and they're not just men.

The idea of purchasing intimacy and paying for the services can be affirming for many people who need human connection, friendship and emotional support. Some people may have fantasies and kink pref- erences that they are able to fulfil with the services of a sex worker. Evidence, not morality, should guide law reforms and sex work policy for full sex work decriminalisation. Sex work is real work.

LGBTQIA+

We live in a society where heterosexuality is assumed for certain people and the assumptions, often prejudiced and unfair, about those who identify within the LGBTQIA+ umbrella continue to be prevalent. Assumptions are still made, for example, that a woman married to a man is heterosexual or that a queer couple have no plans to have children. These assumptions are not only on an individual level however, even the legislations that speak to same-sex couple marriage and child adoptions by queer families are a form of discrimination.

Hate crimes against black lesbian women resulting in rape and murder, as currently experienced in South Africa, requires urgent specialised investigation and prosecution, which is yet to be committed. When these horrendous crimes are under-reported and when urgent and holistic survivor support is non-existent, with neither recourse nor justice tangible, we cannot continue to ignore these human rights violations.

My weekly sexual health column in *The Sunday Times* remains an exciting feature in my career. Week after week, I get to answer questions from readers, which means not only is the column varied in its themes but it is also interesting to see the issues that move people. The usual questions about penis size, length and how many rounds a man can do a night, always feature, so too does the issue of vaginal health and grooming.

I have also written many columns dealing with LGBTQIA+ themed questions, a very welcome surprise. These letters are mainly from parents asking about ways to support their children, teachers asking about providing more affirming curricula and how to best understand the different gender and sexual identities and expression. The LGBTQIA+ community not only has to deal with the marginality that results from being a gender and sexual minority, they too experience the intersections and vulnerabilities of being differently abled and using mobility, visual or audio aids, being a black lesbian woman, being physically located in the peri-urban and rural areas, being an undocumented migrant, a low skilled worker or a sex worker.

It does not matter if you are a black lesbian woman, a transgender woman who is a sex worker, a transgender man who requires a pap smear, or a queer man who has no access to PrEP, the hostile society, discriminating work environments, inaccessible affirming healthcare and prejudice that still exists in some of the laws means that as a society we have no choice but to question what our allyship means as individuals but also what a systemic and structural mandate looks like to ensure human rights of all people need to be protected and promoted.

We must commit to ensuring the thriving of all LGBTQIA+ individuals and this demands resourced action plans at all structures and levels of local governance and diplomatic work on global spaces. We all have to start where we are and through my organisation, Nalane for Reproductive Justice, a group of individuals; some of us are great at research, others in resource mobilising, cross-movement building, facilitating, writing, advocacy, law and clinical services, we continue to advocate for a deliberate and resourced shift to centre those whose gender and sexual identities continue to deem them marginalised, and at the bottom of the ladder for social, economic, sexual, reproductive and gender justice.

A glossary with a difference

···

Acronyms, terms and their definitions are forever evolving. Never more so in the area of sexual health, wellness, pleasure, identity, gender, rights. And the list goes on! Language gives meaning to words and to meaning we attach ideas and emotions and those inform our outlook on life. It is important to remember that over the years many words have evolved in their meaning and use and thus the glossary below represents words and meanings which may mean different things to different people. The list is not exhaustive and aims to provide the basics to form points for discussion and understanding.

Ableism: The pervasive system of discrimination and exclusion that oppresses people who have mental, emotional and physical disabilities.

Abortion: A medical procedure that ends a pregnancy. There are two types of abortions: surgical and medical. Surgical abortions utilise a procedure called vacuum aspiration. Medical abortions, also called drug-induced abortions, involve taking medication that terminates a pregnancy.

Abortion provider: The place where a person can get an abortion, or the healthcare professional who performs the abortion. Examples could include a government clinic or hospital, a private doctor, or a private clinic.

Abstinence: This word means not doing something. It is most commonly used to describe not engaging in sexual activities. Each person decides which activities they include in their definition of abstinence. A person who practices sexual abstinence may say that they are 'abstinent', and what qualifies as being abstinent from sexual activities can vary from person to person (for example abstinent from penetrative sex but not masturbation).

Abstinence-only education: A form of sexual education that teaches only about abstinence. No information is provided about other topics such as consent or safer sex practices such as condoms or contraceptives.

Advocate:
(Noun) Someone who calls attention to a social problem and asks people with authority (lawmakers, school board members, etc.) to address that problem.
(Verb) To call attention to a social problem and to work actively towards a positive change that addresses that problem.

AFAB/AMAB: Acronyms meaning 'assigned female at birth' or 'assigned male at birth'. No one, whether cis or trans, gets to choose what sex they're assigned at birth. We use this term instead of 'biological sex' or 'born as a boy/girl'.

Age of consent: The age when a person is legally able to consent to sexual activities.

Ageism: Any attitude, action, or institutional structure, which subordinates a person or group because of age or any assignment of roles in society purely on the basis of age.

Allosexism: The pervasive system of discrimination and exclusion that oppresses asexual people.

Allosexual: A sexual orientation generally characterised by feeling sexual attraction or a desire for partnered sexuality.

Ally: Someone who is not a member of a group that tends to be discriminated against (such as people who identify as LGBTQIA+), but who works to support members of that group.

Allyship: The action of working to end oppression through support of, and as an advocate with, and for, a group other than one's own.

Anal play: A sexual behaviour where the anal area is stimulated for sexual pleasure, with or without penetration.

Analingus: A sexual act where a person's mouth and/or tongue is used to stimulate the anal zone. This is also known as rimming.

Androgynous: Identifying and/or presenting as neither distinguishably masculine nor feminine. It can refer to things like clothing or gender identity.

Anti-choice: Someone who does not support a person's right to decide whether or not to have an abortion.

Aromantic: A romantic orientation generally characterised by not feeling romantic attraction or a desire for romance. Aromantic people can be satisfied by friendship and other non-romantic relationships.

Arousal: The changes in the body that occur as a result of sexual excitement. These include an erection, vaginal lubrication and an increased sense of sexual awareness.

Asexual: A sexual orientation generally characterised by not feeling sexual attraction or a desire for partnered sexuality. Asexuality is distinct from celibacy, which is the deliberate abstention from sexual activity. Some asexual people do have sex. There are many diverse ways of being asexual.

Bacterial vaginosis: Also known as 'BV', one of the most common vaginal condition in people with vaginas. It is sometimes accompanied by discharge, odour, pain or burning.

Barrier method: Contraceptive methods that protect against pregnancy by placing a physical barrier between sperm and egg. This includes condoms (internal and external), diaphragms, and the sponge. Some barrier methods protect against the transmission of STIs (condoms) others do not (diaphragm).

BDSM: Bondage and Discipline, Dominance and Submission, Sadism and Masochism. BDSM refers to a wide spectrum of activities and forms of interpersonal relationships. While not always overtly sexual in nature, the activities and relationships within a BDSM context are almost always eroticised.

Bi-curious: A term that refers to someone who is primarily attracted to people of one gender, but who has romantic or sexual thoughts about people of another gender.

Biromantic: A person who is romantically attracted to at least one other gender. This is different from being bisexual because it's a romantic orientation, not a sexual orientation.

Bisexual: A person whose primary sexual and affectional orientation is towards people of the same and other genders, or towards people regardless of their gender.

Blowjob: Also called 'giving head'; this is slang for oral sex on a penis.

Body image: Refers to how a person feels, acts, and thinks about their body. Attitudes about our own body and bodies in general are shaped by our communities, families, cultures, media, and our own perceptions.

Body policing: Any behaviour which (indirectly or directly, intentionally or unintentionally) attempts to correct or control a person's actions regarding their own physical body, frequently with regards to gender expression or size.

Butch: An LGBTQIA+ gender expression that leans towards masculinity. Although commonly associated with masculine queer or lesbian women, it is used by many to describe a distinct gender identity or expression, and does not necessarily imply that one also identifies as a woman.

Cisgender: A gender identity, or performance in a gender role, that society deems to match the person's assigned sex at birth. The prefix 'cis-' means 'on this side of' or 'not across'. A term used to call attention to the privilege of people who are not transgender.

Cissexism/Genderism: The pervasive system of discrimination and exclusion that oppresses people whose gender and/or gender expression falls outside of cis-normative constructs. This system is founded on the belief that there are, and should be, only two genders and that one's gender or most aspects of it, are inevitably tied to assigned sex. Within cissexism, cisgender people are the dominant/agent group and trans/gender non-conforming people are the oppressed/target group.

Coming out: 'Coming out' describes voluntarily making public one's sexual orientation and/or gender identity. It has also been broadened to include other pieces of potentially stigmatised personal information. Terms also used that correlate with this action are: 'Being out' which means not concealing one's sexual orientation or gender identity, and 'Outing', a term used for making public the sexual orientation or gender identity of another who would prefer to keep this information secret.

Comprehensive sex education: A type of educational content that adopts a positive view of sexuality as it is a natural part of human development. It provides information about bodily functions, consent, as well as pregnancy and STI prevention, and provides people with skills to make decisions about how to take care of themselves by making informed decisions.

Consent: When a person agrees to a certain action or activity. A person, in order to consent, must have the capacity to consent, which means they are not under the influence of drugs or alcohol, and are of legal age to be able to consent.

Contraceptive: A collection of methods that are used to prevent pregnancy.

Cross-dresser (CD): A word to describe a person who occasionally wears clothes, make-up, and accessories culturally associated with women for example, as a man, and carries no implications of sexual orientation.

Culture: A learnt set of values, beliefs, customs, norms, and perceptions shared by a group of people that provide a general design for living and a pattern for interpreting life.

Cunnilingus: A sexual activity where oral sex is performed on a vulva, including the clitoris and vagina.

Demisexual: Demisexuality is a sexual orientation in which someone feels sexual attraction only to people with whom they have an emotional bond. Most demisexuals feel sexual attraction rarely compared to the general population, and some have little to no interest in sexual activity. Demisexuals are considered to be on the asexual spectrum, meaning they are closely aligned with asexuality.

Dental dam: A thin square of latex used to cover the vulva during oral sex or the anus during sexual play to reduce the risk of the spreading of STIs.

Dildo: A penis-shaped sex toy often made of rubber, silicone, or plastic.

Discrimination: Inequitable actions carried out by members of a dominant group or its representatives against members of a marginalised or minoritised group.

Dry sex: A sexual acts that encompasses going through the motions of sex, ,rubbing fully-clothed bodies, especially genitals against each other. It is also called 'dry humping'.

External condom: An external condom is a thin covering, usually made of latex rubber, that is worn over an erect (hard) penis or sex toy during oral, vaginal or anal sex.

Fellatio: The clinical term for oral sex on a penis.

Femme: Historically used in the lesbian community, it is being increasingly used by other LGBTQIA+ people to describe gender expressions that reclaim/claim and/or disrupt traditional constructs of femininity.

Fertile: The ability to produce offspring; the ability to get pregnant.

Fingering: Slang for using one or several fingers for sexual play involving the vagina, usually including a combination of touching or rubbing the clitoris and placing fingers inside the vagina.

Foetus: An organism that develops from an embryo after about eight weeks of pregnancy. A foetus receives nourishment through the placenta. It will eventually develop to full term and when it is born is called a baby.

Foreplay: All of the sexual activities, stimulation that people might do to get each other sexually aroused (or turned on).

G-spot: This is short for the 'Gräfenberg' spot (named after a gynaecologist) inside the vagina that can produce intense sexual pleasure in some people when stimulated.

Gay: A sexual and affectional orientation towards people of the same gender.

Gender: A social construct used to classify a person as a man, woman or some other identity fundamentally different from the sex one is assigned at birth.

Gender expansive: An umbrella term used for individuals who broaden their own culture's commonly held definitions of gender, including expectations for its expression, identities, roles, and/or other perceived gender norms. Gender expansive individuals include those who identify as transgender, as well as anyone else whose gender in some way is seen to be stretching the surrounding society's notion of gender.

Gender expression: How one expresses oneself in terms of dress and/or behaviours. Society, and people that make up society, characterise these expressions as 'masculine', 'feminine', or 'androgynous'. Individuals may embody their gender in a multitude of ways and have terms beyond these to name their gender expression(s).

Gender fluid: A person whose gender identification and presentation shifts, whether within or outside of societal, gender-based expectations. Being fluid in motion between two or more genders.

Gender identity: A sense of one's self as transgender, gender queer, woman, man or some other identity, which may or may not correspond with the sex and gender one is assigned at birth.

Genderism/Cissexism: Is the belief that there are, and should be, only two genders and that one's gender, or most aspects of it are inevitably tied to assigned sex. In a genderist/cissexist construct, cisgender people are the dominant/agent group and trans/gender non-conforming people are the oppressed/target group.

Gender non-conforming (GNC): People who do not subscribe to gender expressions or roles expected of them by society.

Gender outlaw: A person who refuses to be defined by conventional definitions of male and female.

Gender queer: A person whose gender identity and/or gender expression falls outside of the dominant societal norm for their assigned sex, is beyond genders, or is some combination of them.

Gender variant: A person who varies from the expected characteristics of the assigned gender.

Harassment: Any unwelcome or offensive behaviour by one person to another. Examples are bullying, unwanted, ongoing sexual attention, threats and intimidation.

Heteronormativity: A set of lifestyle norms, practices, and institutions that promote binary alignment of biological sex, gender identity and gender roles; assume heterosexuality as a fundamental and natural norm; and privilege monogamous, committed relationships and reproductive sex above all other sexual practices.

Heterosexism: The assumption that all people are or should be heterosexual. Heterosexism excludes the needs, concerns, and life experiences of lesbian, gay, bisexual and queer people while it gives advantages to heterosexual people. It is often a subtle form of oppression, which reinforces realities of silence and erasure.

Heterosexuality: A sexual orientation in which a person feels physically and emotionally attracted to people of a gender other than their own.

Homosexual/Homosexuality: An outdated term to describe a sexual orientation in which a person feels physically and emotionally attracted to people of the same gender. Historically, it was a term used to pathologise gay and lesbian people.

Internal condom: This is a soft, loose fitting, non-latex pouch that lines the inside of the vagina or anus during sex. Internal condoms should not be used at the same time as external condoms.

Internalised oppression: The fear and self-hate of one's own target/subordinate identity/ies, that occurs for many individuals who have learnt negative ideas about their target/subordinate identity/ies throughout life. One form of internalised oppression is the acceptance of the myths and stereotypes applied to the oppressed group.

Intersex: Adjective used to describe the experience of naturally (that is, without any medical intervention) developing primary or secondary sex characteristics that do not fit neatly into society's definitions of male or female. Intersex is an umbrella term and there are around 20 variations of intersex that are included in this umbrella term. Many visibly Intersex people are mutilated in infancy and early childhood by doctors, to make the individual's sex characteristics conform to society's idea of what normal bodies should look like. Intersex people are relatively common, although society's denial of their existence has allowed very little room for intersex issues to be discussed publicly. Hermaphrodite is an outdated and inaccurate term that has been used to describe intersex people in the past.

Invisibility: Because straight and cis cultures are assumed to be what's normal and LGBTQIA+ identities and experiences are 'other', LGBTQIA+ people are not always seen or represented. This is why LGBTQIA+ people have to continue to come out. If they didn't, they would be assumed to be straight or cis.

Kink: (Kinky, Kinkiness) Most commonly referred to as unconventional sexual practices from which people derive varying forms of pleasure and consensually play-out various forms of desire, fantasies and scenes.

Lesbian: A woman whose primary sexual and affectional orientation is towards people of the same gender.

LGBT: Abbreviation for Lesbian, Gay, Bisexual and Transgender. An umbrella term that is often used to refer to the community as a whole. Our centre uses LGBTQIA+ to intentionally include and raise awareness of Queer, Intersex and Asexual as well as myriad other communities under our umbrella.

LGBTQIA+ allyship: The practice of confronting heterosexism, sexism, genderism, allosexism, and monosexism in oneself and others out of self-interest and a concern for the well-being of lesbian, gay, bisexual, transgender, queer, intersex and asexual people. It believes that dismantling heterosexism, monosexism, trans oppression/trans misogyny/cissexism and allosexism is a social justice issue.

Lubricant: A substance that reduces chafing, irritation and discomfort during many types of sexual activities.

Masturbation: The touching of one's own body, especially the genitals, for sexual pleasure.

Microaggressions: Brief and commonplace daily verbal, behavioural, or environmental indignities, whether intentional or unintentional, that communicate hostile, derogatory, or negative slights and insults about one's marginalised identity/identities.

Misgendering: Attributing a gender to someone that is incorrect or does not align with their gender identity. Can occur when using pronouns, gendered language or assigning genders to people without knowing how they identify.

Monogamy: Having only one intimate partner at any one time.

Monosexism: The belief in and systematic privileging of monosexuality as superior, and the systematic oppression of non-monosexuality.

Monosexual: People who have romantic, sexual, or affectional desire for one gender only. Heterosexuality and homosexuality are the most well-known forms of monosexuality.

MSM: An abbreviation for men who have sex with men; they may or may not identify as gay.

Mutual masturbation: When people either touch their own genitals while they are together, or touch each others' genitals at the same time for sexual pleasure.

Non-binary: A gender identity and experience that embraces a full universe of expressions and ways of being that resonate for an individual. It may be an active resistance to binary gender expectations and/or an intentional creation of new unbounded ideas of self within the world. For some people who identify as non-binary there may be overlap with other concepts and identities like gender expansive and gender non-conforming.

Non-monogamy: A type of relationship style where partners are free to be involved with more than one person at once.

Orientation: Orientation is one's attraction or non-attraction to other people. An individual's orientation can be fluid and people use a variety of labels to describe their orientation. Some, but not all, types of attraction or orientation include: romantic, sexual, sensual, aesthetic, intellectual and platonic.

Pansexual/Omnisexual: Terms used to describe people who have romantic, sexual or affectional desire for people of all genders and sexes.

PEP: Stands for Post-exposure prophylaxis, antiretroviral (ARV) medication taken for a period of time to prevent HIV infection after a recent possible exposure to the virus.

Phobia: In terms of mental/emotional wellness, a phobia is an arced and persistent fear 'out of proportion' to the actual threat or danger the situation poses, after taking into account all the factors of the environment and situation. Historically this term has been used to inaccurately refer to systems oppression (i.e. homophobia has been used to refer to heterosexism). As staff, we've been intentionally moving away from using words like 'transphobic', 'homophobic', and 'biphobic' because (1) they inaccurately describe systems of oppression as irrational fears and (2) for some people, phobias are a very distressing part of their lived experience and co-opting this language is disrespectful to their experiences and perpetuates ableism.

Platonic: A term to describe a relationship that does not include romance or sex; a non-sexual friendship.

Polyamory: Denotes consensually being in/open to multiple loving relationships at the same time. Some polyamorists (polyamorous people) consider 'polyam' to be a relationship orientation. Sometimes used as an umbrella term for all forms of ethical, consensual and loving non-monogamy.

Polygender/Pangender: Exhibiting characteristics of multiple genders, deliberately refuting the concept of only two genders.

Pornography: Books, magazines, movies, and videos about sexually related topics that are designed to cause arousal in the people who read or view them. What can be considered pornography (as opposed to erotic literature or art) varies considerably.

PrEP: Stands for pre-exposure prophylaxis, an ARV pill taken daily that can help prevent HIV.

Pro-choice: A point of view that supports a person's right to decide whether to carry a pregnancy to term or to have an abortion.

Pronouns: Linguistic tools used to refer to someone in the third person. Examples are they/them/theirs, ze/hir/hirs, she/her/hers, he/him/his. In English and some other languages, pronouns have been tied to gender and are a common site of misgendering (attributing a gender to someone that is incorrect).

Queer: Historically, queer has been used as an epithet/slur against people whose gender, gender expression and/or sexuality do not conform to dominant expectations. Some people have reclaimed the word queer and self identify as such. For some, this reclamation is a celebration of not fitting into norms/being 'abnormal'. Manifestations of oppression within gay and lesbian movements such as racism, sizeism, ableism, cissexism, transmisogyny as well as assimilation politics, resulted in many people being marginalised, thus, for some, queer is a radical and anti-assimilationist stance that captures multiple aspects of identities.

Questioning: The process of exploring one's own gender identity, gender expression, and/or sexual orientation. Some people may also use this term to name their identity within the LGBTQIA+ community.

Romantic orientation: Romantic Orientation is attraction or non-attraction to other people characterised by the expression or non-expression of love. Romantic orientation can be fluid and people use a variety of labels to describe their romantic orientation. See also **Orientation**.

Sex: A medically constructed categorisation. Sex is often assigned based on the appearance of the external genitalia at birth.

Sex negativity: Dislike or hostility towards open expressions of sexuality.

Sex positivity: An attitude that says that consensual and pleasurable sexual activities are healthy, including the decision not to have sex at all.

Sexism: Discrimination based on biological sex or gender, specifically discrimination against women. These are attitudes, conditions, or behaviours that promote stereotyping of social roles based on real or perceived gender.

Sexuality: Sexuality is a broad term that refers to far more than sexual activities and body parts. The components of a person that include their biological sex, sexual orientation and gender identity.

Sexual orientation: Sexual orientation is an enduring emotional, romantic, sexual or affectional attraction or non-attraction to other people. Sexual orientation can be fluid and people use a variety of labels to describe their sexual orientation.

Spooning: When two people lie on their sides, both facing the same direction, and either wrap their arms around each other for intimacy or to sleep, or as a position for sexual intercourse.

Swinger (Swinging): A person or people in a committed relationship consensually engaging in sexual activity with others.

Trans man: A person may choose to identify this way to capture their gender identity as well as their lived experience as a transgender person. Some trans men may also use the term FTM or F2M to describe their identity.

Trans woman: A person may choose to identify this way to capture their gender identity as well as their lived experience as a transgender person. Some trans women may also use MTF or M2F to describe their identity.

Transgender: Adjective used most often as an umbrella term, and frequently abbreviated to 'trans'. This adjective describes a wide range of identities and experiences of people whose gender identity and/or expression differs from conventional expectations based on their assigned sex at birth. Not all trans people undergo medical transition (surgery or hormones).

Transition: An individualised process by which transgender people move from one gender presentation to another. There are three general aspects to transitioning: social (i.e. name, pronouns, interactions, etc.), medical (i.e. hormones, surgery, etc.), and legal (i.e. gender marker and name change, etc.). A trans individual may transition in any combination, or none, of these aspects.

Vibrator: A battery or electrically powered device used to massage and provide stimulation to the body, especially the genitals.

Womxn: Some womxn spell the word with an 'x' as a form of empowerment to move away from the 'men' in the 'traditional' spelling of women.

WSW: An abbreviation for women who have sex with women; they may or may not identify as lesbian.

Zie/Hir: Alternate pronouns that are gender neutral and preferred by some gender non-conforming people. Pronounced 'zee' and 'here', they replace 'he'/'she' and 'his'/'hers' respectively.

Health and wellness checklist

....

Each decade that passes adds onto the screening tests and lifestyle advice from the previous decade, taking into consideration individual needs, risks and management options. Mental health is an important part of wellness and seeking therapy and medical advice for mental illness must be encouraged. The best advice, generally, is to know your body and recognise any unexpected or abnormal changes and seek advice from your healthcare provider.

In your 20s

It may not feel like it now but your body is going to require some attention to ensure health and longevity. Exercise will help with strengthening your bones and promoting a healthy cardiovascular system and keeping the kegels, the pelvic floor muscles, healthy.

Well-woman visit

Go for annual check-ups that include skin examination, a breast exam and tips on how to perform a self-breast exam, a pelvic exam and tips on how to check your vulva, STI screening tests and your first pap smear. This will include a discussion on contraception choices, sexual pleasure and STI prevention.

Dental and optician visit

Taking care of your teeth and eyes is so, so important and you therefore need to make annual visits to the dentist and optician. You are never 'too young' and might find you may even need to make use of assisted visual aids such as glasses.

Blood pressure screening

Know your family history of hypertension. Use of the combined oral contraceptive pill will help determine your risks and how often you need to check your blood pressure. Simple lifestyle changes, such as exercising and eating a well-balanced diet, may be sufficient for you.

Cholesterol screening

If you have a personal history of coronary artery disease, tobacco use, high blood pressure or obesity, seeking advice and early intervention is important.

Vaccination

The tetanus vaccine booster is recommended once every 10 years and with advice during pregnancy.

In your 30s

This is the time to focus on building on your foundation for good health and to address health concerns. You may feel agile and strong but your body is starting to age.

Well-woman visit

A regular pap smear with HPV testing is recommended. A discussion with your healthcare provider about reproductive issues, fertility, assisted fertility options available and relationship advice are all topics that should be covered.

Nutritious diet

Hair, nails and skin health are all partly impacted by diet. Bone, cholesterol, joint and muscle health, as well as cardiovascular and mental health concerns will inform your choices about diet and supplements.

Skincare

Sun exposure over the years may result in hyperpigmentation or even cancer. It's never too late to use sunscreen! Fine lines appearing around the lips and on the cheeks may be due to smoking. A receding hairline from damage due to chemicals and hairstyles can start.

Mental health

Identify and seek medical advice for any behavioural concerns such as mood changes, cognitive changes such as memory, concentration changes, eating or sleeping pattern changes and the use of substances and substance abuse.

In your 40s

You may become so focused on the balance between life, work and family but do not neglect your health in the process! This is also the time when the benefits of healthy habits of yesteryears come to fruition. Many lifestyle risks such as diabetes, cholesterol and cancers become diseases and illnesses in your forties.

Well-woman visit

The frequency and screening tests done during your well-woman visit may change based on past test results. It is important to remember that it is never too late to start annual well-woman visits.

Bone health

A bone density scan to monitor the health of your bones may be recommended, especially if you have a history of using Depo-Provera injectable contraceptive.

Breast health

A mammogram may be advised at this age. As with many screening tests, the appropriateness is based on your individual risk factors and family history. An ultrasound of the breasts may also be performed.

Reproductive health

Your menstrual cycle might start to change and a discussion about the symptoms of menopause is important. Reviewing contraceptive options and their effectiveness and appropriateness is useful at this stage.

In your 50s

At this point, you may be on medication for a chronic illness. Or the lifestyle and preventive healthcare changes made in earlier years, will continue to pay off. You might start to have more regular tests and checks done during this decade.

Bone health

Once menopause starts, bone density begins to decrease as your body produces less oestrogen. A bone density scan to monitor the health of the bones, especially if you have a family history of osteoporosis is advised.

Chronic disease

Management of conditions such as diabetes, hypertension, mental illness or obesity may take some dedication and getting used to. You may be on hormone replacement therapy post-menopause.

Breast health

A mammogram and ultrasound of the breasts is recommended. Some are scheduled every two years starting from age 50 to help in early detection of breast cancer.

Colorectal screening

A colonoscopy is the most effective screening tool and the recommendation from your healthcare provider will suit your particular circumstances in terms of polyps and cancer.

Vaccinations

Boosters as well as new vaccinations may be recommended with pneumococcal and influenza some of the more common vaccinations recommend on an annual basis.

In your 60s

With age, the risk of developing some cancers increases. It is never too late to stop smoking and exercise in any form is good for your cardio-vascular system, bone health and mental health.

Mental health

Learning new skills, doing puzzles or crosswords, reading and socialising keeps the brain healthy. Diseases such as dementia are common as one gets older.

Visit to the optician

Screen for vision, mobility or cognitive issues that might impact your ability to be a safe driver.

Acknowledgements

Having words is great, and I have plenty to say, but turning those words into a book is not easy. This experience has been challenging and rewarding all at the same time. I especially want to thank the entire Pan Macmillan family: Terry, Jane, Sandile, Karel and Andrea, all of whom I have worked closely with, as well as the rest of the team who helped to make this book happen with all their behind-the-scenes work.

To my mother: Agnes 'Ausi Aggie' Matjele-Mofokeng, not only did you nurture me and provide me with the best childhood and support to pursue my dreams, but you are also a friend, a mentor and a continuous source of inspiration. Thank you for teaching me discipline, unconditional love and how to remain excited with life every day. I truly have no idea where I'd be if you were not my mother. Thank you for raising my son so that I can gallivant the world over and be amazing.

To my life partner: Lacks, thank you for taking care of me. When I forgot to eat and stay hydrated while writing, you were always on cue. You put up with a lot, truly you do, and I really appreciate your kindness and love. Sox! ☺

Bukhosibemvelo: Son, ngwanaka, you are the most exquisite thing I have ever experienced and I love you so much. Thank you for always calling to tell me how beautiful I am on TV, or that you heard my voice on the radio. You're the cutest cheerleader. By the time this book goes to print, I will still be on the mzabalazo for land, but I do promise you that this world will be a much better place for you and all the children in the world to thrive. I will do everything to ensure that you are filled with pride to point me out in a crowd and call me Mme.

Leano: Bitso wa ka, thank you for being such an amazing companion and friend to MaV. You make me proud in so many ways. And to Neo, Letlotlo, Arya, Queen, Tshepo, one of the greatest privileges is to be your aunt. I love watching you grow.

My brothers: Nkejane, Pheello, Teboho, thank you for an amazing archive of memories and joy. I know I generally give you a hard time but I think you expect it now, so just this one time, let me say thank you for putting up with me.

To the women who came before, who anchor and continue to inspire:

Professors Loretta Ross and Kimberle Crenshaw. From across continents, you taught me so much and continue to enrich my life with thought leadership and the scholarship required to navigate this world through the struggles these groups, through identity, life experiences, classism and sexism, endure. Thank you.

Prof Elna McIntosh: Your career was the inspiration for a path I would choose as my life. For many years before we even met, you mentored me without even knowing. You've held my hand, so thank you. The airport drop-offs and pick-ups have defined some of the best times we've had.

To my chosen family, my friendships: Tanya, Letlhogonolo, Mapheko, Kgomotso, Lebo, Nadine (especially for the support with scribing), Janice, Siyophumelela, Edith, Mandisa, Lesego, Seoketsi, Ndu, Dudu, Nomtika.

To everyone who was here for this journey, thank you. I appreciate you.

Selected references

Allen KR, Goldberg AE. Sexual activity during menstruation: a qualitative study. J Sex Res. 2009 Nov–Dec; 46(6): 535–45.

Anderson, F. American Journal of Psychiatry, 2009; vol 166, no 5: pp 591 and 598.

Breuner CC, Mattson G. Sexuality education for children and adolescents. AAP Committee on Adolescence, AAP Committee on Psychosocial Aspects of Child and Family Health. Pediatrics 2016; 138(2).

Carroll NM. Medical care of sexual minority women http://www.uptodate.com/contents/search, accessed September 11, 2017.

Crenshaw K. Demarginalizing the Intersection of Race and Sex: A Black Feminist Critique of Antidiscrimination Doctrine, Feminist Theory and Antiracist Politics, University of Chicago Legal Forum: Vol. 1989: Issue 1, Article 8.

Frumovitz M. Invasive cervical cancer: Epidemiology, risk factors, clinical manifestations, and diagnosis http://www.uptodate.com/home, accessed April 1, 2016.

Gabbe SG, et al., eds. Preconception and prenatal care. In: Obstetrics: Normal and Problem Pregnancies. 7th ed. Philadelphia, Pa.: Elsevier; 2017. http://www.clinicalkey.com. Accessed June 14, 2018.

Gay CL, et al. Prevention of sexually transmitted infections. http://www.uptodate.com/home, accessed July 31, 2016.

Hogarth H, Ingham R. Masturbation among Young Women and Associations with Sexual Health: An Exploratory Study, The Journal of Sex Research, 2009; 46(6): 558–567.

Jensen PT, Froeding LP. Pelvic radiotherapy and sexual function in women. Transl Androl Urol. 2015 Apr 4 (2): 186–205.

Knight DA, et al. Preventive health care for women who have sex with women. American Family Physician. 2017; 95: 314.

Lee R. Health care problems of lesbian, gay, bisexual, and transgender patients. West J Med. 2000; 172(6): 403–408.

Lentz GM, et al. Infections of the lower and upper genital tracts. In: Comprehensive Gynecology. 6th ed. Philadelphia, Pa.: Mosby Elsevier; 2012.

http://www.clinicalkey.com, accessed January 18, 2016.

Longo DL, et al., eds. Human immunodeficiency virus disease: AIDS and related disorders. In: Harrison's Principles of Internal Medicine. 19th ed. New York, N.Y.: McGraw-Hill Education; 2015.

Mazokopakis EE, Samonis G. Is Vaginal Sexual Intercourse Permitted during Menstruation? A Biblical (Christian) and Medical Approach. Maedica (Buchar). 2018; 13(3): 183–188.

Ngabaza S, Shefer T, Macleod CI. (2016). Girls need to behave like girls you know: the complexities of applying a gender justice goal within sexuality education in South African schools. Reproductive Health Matters, 1–8.

Niederhuber JE, et al., eds. Cancers of the cervix, vulva, and vagina. In: Abeloff's Clinical Oncology. 5th ed. Philadelphia, Pa.: Churchill Livingstone Elsevier; 2014 http://www.clinicalkey.com, accessed April 1, 2016.

Olson KR, et al. Mental health of transgender children who are supported in their identities. Pediatrics 2015; 137(1).

Olson-Kennedy J, et al. Overview of the management of gender nonconformity in children and adolescents. http://www.uptodate.com/contents/search, accessed December 23, 2016.

Parker, RG. Sexuality, health, and human rights. Am J Public Health. 2007; 97(6): 972–973.

Rimal, RN, Lapinski, MK. Bulletin of the World Health Organization 2009; 87: 24–247.

Ross LJ. Reproductive Justice as Intersectional Feminist Activism, Souls, 2017 19:3, 286–314.

Shefer T, Kruger L, Macleod C, Baxen J, Vincent L (2015) '… a huge monster that should be feared and not done': Lessons learned in sexuality education classes in South Africa. African Safety Promotion: A Journal of Injury and Violence Prevention, 13 (1), 71–86.

Shefer T, Macleod C. (2015) Life Orientation sexuality education in South Africa: Gendered norms, justice and transformation. Perspectives in Education, 33 (2), 1–10.

Shifren JL, Johannes CB, Monz BU, Russo PA, Bennett L, Rosen R. Help-seeking behavior of women with self-reported distressing sexual problems. J Women's Health 2009; 18: 461–468.

Sobel JD. Approach to women with symptoms of vaginitis. http://www.uptodate.com/contents/search, accessed February 7, 2019.

Spatz ES, et al. Sexual activity and function among middle-aged and older men and women with hypertension. Journal of Hypertension. 2013; 31:1.

Unger CA. Hormone therapy for transgender patients. Transl Androl Urol. 2016; 5(6): 877–884.

Unger CA, Marecek J, Macleod C, Hoggart L (2017). Abortion in legal, social, and healthcare contexts. Feminism & Psychology, 27(1), 4–14.

Ussher JM, Perz J, Gilbert E. Perceived causes and consequences of sexual changes after cancer for women and men: a mixed method study. BMC Cancer. 2015; Apr 11; 15: 268.

Wein AJ, et al., eds. Evaluation and management of erectile dysfunction. In:

Campbell-Walsh Urology. 10th ed. Philadelphia, Pa.: Elsevier Saunders; 2012. http://www.clinicalkey.com, accessed July 8, 2015.

Other sources

An adapted version of the OpenStax Anatomy & Physiology with revised content and artwork.

Anatomy and Physiology by Openstax Pub Date: 2013, http://library.open.oregonstate.edu/aandp/.

Birth control methods. Office on Women's Health. https://www.womenshealth.gov/a-z-topics/birth-control-methods, accessed August 9, 2017.

Comprehensive sexuality education. Committee Opinion No. 678. American College of Obstetricians and Gynecologists. Obstet Gynecol 2016; 128:e227-30

Diabetes and female sexuality. (2015) my.clevelandclinic.org/health/articles/7826-diabetes-and-female-sexuality.

Diabetes and sexual and urological problems. (2018) niddk.nih.gov/health-information/diabetes/overview/preventing-problems/sexual-bladder-problems.

Frequently asked questions. Pregnancy FAQ090. Early pregnancy loss. American College of Obstetricians and Gynecologists. https://www.acog.org/Patients/FAQs/Early-Pregnancy-Loss, accessed June 14, 2018.

Frequently asked questions. Women's health FAQ190. Vulvovaginal health. American College of Obstetricians and Gynecologists. http://www.acog.org/Patients/FAQs/Vulvovaginal-Health, accessed February 7, 2019.

HIV treatment as prevention. HIV.gov. https://www.hiv.gov/hiv-basics/hiv-prevention/using-hiv-medication-to-reduce-risk/hiv-treatment-as-prevention, accessed December 15, 2017.

Information for teens and young adults: Staying healthy and preventing STDs. US Centers for Disease Control and Prevention. http://www.cdc.gov/std/life-stages-populations/stdfact-teens.htm, accessed July 31, 2016.

Lesbian and bisexual health. The National Women's Health Information Center. https://www.womenshealth.gov/a-z-topics/lesbian-and-bisexual-health, accessed September 11, 2017.

McGraw-Hill Education; 2015. http://accessmedicine.mhmedical.com, accessed Dec 15, 2017.

Overview of sexually transmitted diseases. Merck Manual Professional Version. http://www.merckmanuals.com/professional/infectious-diseases/sexually-transmitted-diseases-std/overview-of-sexually-transmitted-diseases. Accessed Dec 6, 2015.

PrEP. Centers for Disease Control and Prevention. https://www.cdc.gov/hiv/basics/prep.html, accessed March 22, 2019.

Sex and high blood pressure. http://www.heart.org/HEARTORG/Conditions/HighBloodPressure/WhyBloodPressureMatters/Sex-and-High-Blood-Pressure_UCM_451787_Article.jsp, accessed September 22, 2015.

Sexual difficulties. U.S. Department of Health and Human Services Office on

Women's Health. http://womenshealth.gov/aging/sexual-health/sexual-diffi-
culties.html, accessed July 26, 2016.

Sexuality in later life. National Institute on Aging. https://www.nia.nih.gov/
health/publication/sexuality-later-life, accessed July 26, 2016.

Sexually transmitted infections (STIs). World Health Organization. http://www.
who.int/mediacentre/factsheets/fs110/en/, accessed December 6, 2015.

Start the conversation. American Sexual Health Association. http://www.
ashasexualhealth.org/parents/how-to-start-the-conversation, accessed July
9, 2016.

STDs during pregnancy – CDC fact sheet. Centers for Disease Control and
Prevention. http://www.cdc.gov/std/pregnancy/STDFact-Pregnancy.htm,
accessed June 14, 2018.

United Nations Population Fund (UNFPA), Emerging Evidence, Lessons and
Practice in Comprehensive Sexuality Education: A Global Review, Paris:
United Nations Educational, Scientific and Cultural Organization, 2015
https://www.unfpa.org/publications/emerging-evidence-lessons-and-prac-
tice-comprehensive-sexuality-education-global-review; https://openstax.org/
details/anatomy-and-physiology.

What is atherosclerosis? National Heart, Lung, and Blood Institute. http://
www.nhlbi.nih.gov/health/health-topics/topics/atherosclerosis/, accessed
July 8, 2015.

What to do when diabetes affects your sex life. (2014) health.clevelandclinic.
org/when-diabetes-affects-your-sex-life.

Websites consulted and extra reading

All websites active at the time of publication

https://www.acog.org/Clinical-Guidance-and-Publications/Committee-
Opinions/Committee-on-Adolescent-Health-Care/Comprehensive-
Sexuality-Education

https://www.amnesty.org/en/latest/news/2016/05/amnesty-international-pub-
lishes-policy-and-research-on-protection-of-sex-workers-rights/

https://asijiki.org.za

https://www.cosmopolitan.com/sex-love/positions/

https://www.facebook.com/Sex-Talk-With-Dr-T-445816009167963/

http://www.guttmacher.org/fact-sheet/
facts-american-teens-sources-information-about-sex

https://hivlawcommission.org

https://www.independent.ie/irish-news/education/why-teenagers-are-dismiss-
ing-out-of-touch-sex-education-in-irish-schools-35044076.html

https://jamanetwork.com/journals/jamapediatrics/fullarticle/1791584

https://lgbtqia.ucdavis.edu/educated/glossary

http://www.ncbi.nlm.nih.gov/pmc/articles/PMC1874191/

https://www.ncbi.nlm.nih.gov/pmc/articles/PMC5182227/

https://www.ncbi.nlm.nih.gov/pmc/articles/PMC6290188/

https://www.ncbi.nlm.nih.gov/pubmed/26816824

https://www.ncbi.nlm.nih.gov/pubmed/25885443

http://www.nswp.org/sites/nswp.org/files/policy_brief_sex_work_as_work_
nswp_-_2017.pdf

https://www.researchgate.net/publication/233749889_Interventions_Using_
New_Digital_Media_to_Improve_Adolescent_Sexual_Health_A_Systematic_
Review

https://www.researchgate.net/
publication/7851169_Private-sector_caesarean_sections_in_perspective

https://soundcloud.com/user-757075516

https://sugarcookie.com/2014/10/top-5-sex-positions/

http://www.sweat.org.za/what-we-do/sisonke/

https://www.tandfonline.com/doi/full/10.1080/10999949.2017.1389634

http://teenhealthsource.com/definitions/

https://www.theguardian.com/world/2014/sep/24/
caesarean-section-south-africa

https://www.thelancet.com

http://themediaonline.co.za/2018/03/what-the-latest-ram-tells-us-about-radio/

https://www.timeslive.co.za/sunday-times/business/2017-09-28-in-four-years-
78-of-south-africans-will-have-internet-access/http://transhealth.ucsf.edu/
trans?page=guidelines-feminizing-therapy

https://www.uberkinky.co.uk/essential-guides/restraint-guides/beginners-guide-
to-rope-bondage.html

https://www.who.int/bulletin/volumes/87/4/08-056713/en/

https://www.who.int/reproductivehealth/topics/sexual_health/sh_definitions/en/

Social and medical resources

Alcoholics Anonymous South Africa
The only requirement for membership is a desire to stop drinking.
- National helpline: 0861 HELPAA (435 722)
- Website: www.aasouthafrica.org.za

CANSA Care Centres and Care Clinics
Provide holistic care and support to you and your loved ones, from the time of diagnosis, through all phases of need.
- Toll-free call centre: 0800 22 66 22
- Email: info@cansa.org.za

DISA Clinic
No doctor's referral needed to visit the clinic.
- Telephone: 011 787 1222/886 2286
- Fax: 086 617 7371
- Email: disa@icon.co.za
- 15 Lebensraum Place, Hurlingham Manor, Sandton
- Website: http://safersex.co.za

Disabled People South Africa (DPSA)
DPSA is a cross-disability, human rights organisation that is run and managed by disabled people. Advocates for human rights in social, political and economic environment.
- Website: www.dpsa.org.za

Family and Marriage Association of South Africa (Famsa)

Famsa supports families through stressful situations. Assistance with divorce, mediation, domestic violence, trauma, grief counselling, etc.
- Telephone: (011) 975-7106/7
- Email: national@famsa.org.za
- Website: www.famsa.org.za

hi4LIFE – Health Information for Life

Trusted health information for the entire family on your mobile phone; a two-way street of communication.
- Website: www.hi4LIFE.co.za

Hub of Loving Action in Africa (HOLAA!)

HOLAA! is a digital space where women and gender non-conforming people of all sexualities can come together and engage through workshops, dialogues, archiving, digital conversations knowledge production, partnerships and awareness building.
- Website: http://holaafrica.org

Intersex South Africa

An organisation established to spread knowledge about intersex, to provide the space for the development of an intersexed voice in southern Africa, and to combat discrimination on grounds of intersex.

LifeLine Southern Africa

24-hour crisis service. Free, confidential counselling for rape, trauma, AIDS and a range of other services.
- National counselling helpline: 0861 322 322
- Website: www.lifeline.org.za
- National Aids helpline: 0800 012 322 and aidshelpline.org.za
- Stop Gender Violence helpline: 0800 150 150

Nalane for Reproductive Justice: (@Nalane4RJ)

Founded by Dr Tlaleng Mofokeng, it employs an intersectional framework that leverages the synergy between communications and advocacy with a focus primarily on sexual and reproductive health,

rights and access.
https://twitter.com/Nalane4RJ?s=17

National Department of Health – Information for Abortion clinics

Address: Thabo Sehume and Struben's Street, Office 518 North Tower,
  Pretoria
- Telephone: 012 395 9034

Dr Tlaleng Mofokeng, SRHR adviser, health communications and advocacy

- Website: www.drtlaleng.com

People Opposed to Woman Abuse (Powa)

Powa is a Gauteng-based organisation offering shelter, counselling
  and legal support to women in abusive relationships, rape survivors,
  survivors of incest.
- Helpline: 083 765 1235
- Website: www.powa.co.za

Police Child Protection Units

The SA Police Service's Family Violence, Child Protection and Sexual
  Offences Unit Special police units investigate violent crimes against
  children and offer specialised services to child victims of crime.
1. Emergency number: 10111
2. Crime Stop: 08600 10111
3. Report cases of child abuse for police investigation: childprotect@
   saps.org.za
4. Website: www.saps.gov.za

Rape Crisis

Rape Crisis Cape Town Trust works to prevent rape, offers healing
  to survivors, and works towards legal steps that will ensure
  perpetrators are brought to justice.
- Counselling lines:
021 447-9762 (Observatory)
021 633 9229 (Athlone)

021 361 9085 (Khayelitsha)
- Website: www.rapecrisis.org.za

SA *Depression and Anxiety Group*

Can assist in locating a psychiatrist, psychologist or GP with special interest in mental health in your area.
- Suicide crisis line: 0800 567 567 or SMS 31393 (8am–8pm, seven days a week)
- Helpline: (011) 262-6396 (8am–8pm, seven days a week)
- Website: www.sadag.org

Stop Gender Abuse

Crisis counselling for women who have been raped or abused, advice and support for people wanting to support women in need of help.
- Toll-free helpline: 0800 150 150
- Website: www.lifelinesa.co.za

Transgender and intersex Africa on Facebook

Aims to support transgender and intersex individuals with safe spaces to debrief and share necessary information.

CPSIA information can be obtained
at www.ICGtesting.com
Printed in the USA
BVHW031918170919
558677BV00002B/150/P

9 781770 106468